Management of
Chronic Viral Hepatitis
Second Edition

Management of Chronic Viral Hepatitis

Second Edition

GRAHAM R FOSTER, PhD, FRCP
Professor of Hepatology
Queen Mary's School of Medicine and Dentistry
Barts and The London NHS Trust
The Royal London Hospital
London, UK

ROBERT D GOLDIN, MD, FRCPATH
Senior Lecturer in Histopathology
Imperial College Faculty of Medicine
and Consultant Histopathologist
Department of Cellular Pathology
St Mary's Hospital
London, UK

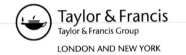
Taylor & Francis
Taylor & Francis Group

LONDON AND NEW YORK

A MARTIN DUNITZ BOOK

© 2002, 2005 Taylor & Francis, an imprint of the Taylor & Francis Group

First published in the UK in 2002
Second edition published by Taylor & Francis, an imprint of the Taylor & Francis Group, 2 Park Square, Milton Park, Abingdon, Oxfordshire, OX14 4RN

Second edition 2005

Tel.:   +44 (0) 20 7017 6000
Fax.:   +44 (0) 20 7017 6699
E-mail: info@dunitz.co.uk
Website: http://www.dunitz.co.uk

Although every effort has been made to ensure that drug doses and other information are presented accurately in this publication, the ultimate responsibility rests with the prescribing physician. Neither the publishers nor the authors can be held responsible for errors or for any consequences arising from the use of information contained herein. For detailed prescribing information or instructions on the use of any product or procedure discussed herein, please consult the prescribing information or instructional material issued by the manufacturer.

A CIP record for this book is available from the British Library.

ISBN 1 84184 479 9

Distributed in North and South America by
Taylor & Francis
2000 NW Corporate Blvd
Boca Raton, FL 33431, USA

Within Continental USA
Tel.: 800 272 7737; Fax.: 800 374 3401
Outside Continental USA
Tel.: 561 994 0555; Fax.: 561 361 6018
E-mail: orders@crcpress.com

Distributed in the rest of the world by
Thomson Publishing Services
Cheriton House
North Way
Andover, Hampshire SP10 5BE, UK
Tel.: +44 (0)1264 332424
E-mail: salesorder.tandf@thomsonpublishingservices.co.uk

Composition by 🡕 TekArt

Printed and bound in Italy by Printer Trento S.r.l.

Contents

Preface

Chronic viral hepatitis affects over 500 million people worldwide and leads to cirrhosis and liver cell cancer in a large proportion of infected individuals. The optimal management of those who are infected requires close collaboration between the pathologist, who identifies the grade and stage of the disease, and the physician who implements therapy.

In this updated edition of this succinct guide, two experienced teachers present a complete guide to the investigation and management of chronic viral hepatitis. The authors outline the mechanisms underlying persistent viral infection and go on to describe the epidemiology, virology and diagnosis of chronic viral hepatitis before outlining a comprehensive guide to modern, biopsy-based management.

This well-written second edition describes the use of the latest therapies, including the pegylated interferons, and will be of value to hepatologists, gastroenterologists and infectious disease physicians who care for patients with chronic viral hepatitis.

Graham R Foster
Robert D Goldin

Abbreviations

AFP	alfa-fetoprotein
AIDS	acquired immunodeficiency syndrome
cccDNA	covalently closed circular DNA
CT	computed tomography
ddI	didanosine
DNA	deoxyribonucleic acid
HAI	histological activity index
HBcAg	hepatitis B virus core antigen
HBeAg	hepatitis B e antigen
HBIg	hepatitis B immunoglobulin
HBsAg	hepatitis B virus surface antigen
HIV	human immunodeficiency virus
HLA	human leucocyte antigen
IL	interleukin
iu	international units
MRI	magnetic resonance imaging
NS	non-structural
PCR	polymerase chain reaction
RNA	ribonucleic acid

Chronic viral hepatitis – persistence, prevalence and transmission

1

Most adult humans suffer from at least four or five viral infections every year. In almost all cases antiviral defence mechanisms recognize and rapidly eliminate the virus so that the illness is usually trivial and short-lasting.

Infection with the chronic hepatotropic viruses is very different – these pathogens commonly evade the antiviral defence systems and cause a long-lasting, persistent infection. The prolonged nature of the infection ensures that every infected person has ample opportunity to transmit the virus to others, allowing many millions of people worldwide to become infected. Three viruses commonly cause chronic hepatitis – hepatitis B virus (HBV), hepatitis C virus (HCV) and the delta virus (HDV). Virologically, these three pathogens are remarkably different but all have developed mechanisms that allow persistent infection, and overall they infect over 500 million people worldwide.

Mechanisms of persistence: how do hepatotropic viruses cause chronic infection?

Most viral infections are transient – after infection the virus is rapidly eliminated by the combined effects of the innate and the acquired immune systems. To cause persistent infection a virus must avoid the host defences, and the hepatotropic viruses have developed elaborate strategies to achieve this.

Avoiding the innate immune system

The innate immune system is the first line of defence against pathogens. It consists of an arsenal of preformed circulating proteins as well as a series of cellular receptors that, when activated, trigger the release of proinflammatory cytokines. The circulating proteins of the innate immune system, such as mannose-binding lectin, bind to and neutralize infecting pathogens. These proteins play a key role in eliminating bacteria but they probably play a relatively minor role in combating viral infection. The surface receptors of the innate system are members of the TOLL-like family of receptors (TLRs). These bind to the products of infectious agents (such as the lipopolysaccharide coat of bacteria) and they activate the release of cytokines, such as tumour necrosis factor (TNF) and interleukin (IL)-1, which lead to inflammation and the activation of macrophages and lymphocytes. Again, activation of the TOLL-like receptors is an important component of the host defence against bacteria, but it is probably only of minor importance in the elimination of viruses.

The most important innate antiviral defence system is the type I interferons. The interferons are a family of closely related cytokines that consists of 12 interferon alpha subtypes, one interferon beta subtype and one interferon omega subtype. These interferons are rapidly produced by virally infected cells and, once released, they bind to cell surface receptors and induce the production of a large number of proteins that inhibit viral replication.

The functions of some of the proteins that are induced by the type I interferons are well characterized, but no function has yet been identified for many of them. Some of the interferon-inducible proteins are produced in an inactive form and are activated by viral products. For example, type I interferons induce the production of a protein kinase known as 'PKR'. In the presence of a replicating RNA virus, this protein is activated by double-stranded RNA, and the activated kinase inhibits cellular protein production, thereby leading to suppression of viral replication. Other interferon-inducible proteins inhibit the replication of other viruses (e.g. the Mx protein inhibits the replication of the influenza virus), and it is assumed that many of the hundred or so interferon-induced proteins identified to date inhibit the replication of specific viruses, although not all of the targets have been identified (Table 1.1). It is not yet known which of the interferon-inducible proteins inhibit the replication of the hepatotropic viruses. The antiviral effects of the type I interferons are shown schematically in Figure 1.1.

In addition to activating an antiviral state in cells exposed to viruses, the type I interferons have immunomodulatory effects. They facilitate immune recognition of virally infected cells by increasing the cell surface expression of the human leucocyte antigen (HLA) class I antigens. These proteins present viral antigens to the cells of the immune system (see page 6) and thereby facilitate the immune-mediated destruction of virally infected cells. The type I interferons also facilitate the activation of the Th1 subset of helper T cells by increasing the expression of the IL-12 receptor and thereby increasing responsiveness to this cytokine.

Since the type I interferons are potent inhibitors of viral replication, viruses that

Table 1.1
Proteins that are induced by interferon alpha. Several hundred proteins are induced when the type I interferons bind to the cell surface receptor, and only a few well-studied examples are listed here.

Protein	Function	Comments
PKR	Inhibits the replication of viruses that contain double-stranded RNA by blocking protein translation	Activated by double-stranded RNA
2′5′ oligoadenylate synthetase	Inhibits the replication of viruses that contain double-stranded RNA by inducing its degradation	Activated by double-stranded RNA
Mx	Inhibits the replication of influenza virus	
HLA class I antigens	Presents foreign peptides to lymphocytes	
IL-12 receptor beta chain	Essential for response to IL-12	Sensitizes naïve T cells to the effects of IL-12 and thereby allows the development of a mature T cell response
6-16	Unknown	Used to study the interferon signal transduction pathway
ISG 15	Unknown	Used to study the interferon signal transduction pathway
9-27	Unknown	
ISG 54	Unknown	

lead to prolonged infection must have developed mechanisms to overcome the effects of these interferons, and many viruses encode proteins that inhibit the interferon system in some way. In the case of the HBV, two proteins are involved in this inhibition – the core protein has been shown to inhibit the production of interferon, and the polymerase protein can inhibit its effects. In the case of the HCV, the core, E2, NS4 and NS5A proteins have all been reported to reduce the effects of interferon in different ways. The core protein may reduce interferon alfa signalling by interfering with the signal transduction pathway at the level of the STAT1 phosphoprotein and the NS5A and E2 proteins can inhibit the antiviral kinase, PKR. Studies with the HCV NS4 protein show that this protein can reduce interferon alfa production by inhibiting the function of the signalling protein IRF3. Hence, like HBV, HCV has developed mechanisms that reduce both the production of, and response to, interferon alfa. However, the clinical relevance of these inhibitory

Figure 1.1
Antiviral effects of the type I interferons. (A) The type I interferon (usually interferon alpha or interferon-beta) binds to the two components of the interferon receptor. (B) Binding and dimerization activates a complex signal transduction pathway that involves sequential activation of a series of phosphoproteins (known as the JAKs and STATs). (C) This process ultimately leads to the induction of a large number of interferon-inducible genes, including Mx, 2'5' oligoadenylate synthetase and the protein kinase PKR. (D) The PKR protein is produced in an inactive form and is activated by double-stranded RNA produced by infecting viruses. (E) The activated kinase inhibits protein translation (by phosphorylating the translation initiation factor eIF2-alpha. The inhibition of protein translation prevents further viral replication.

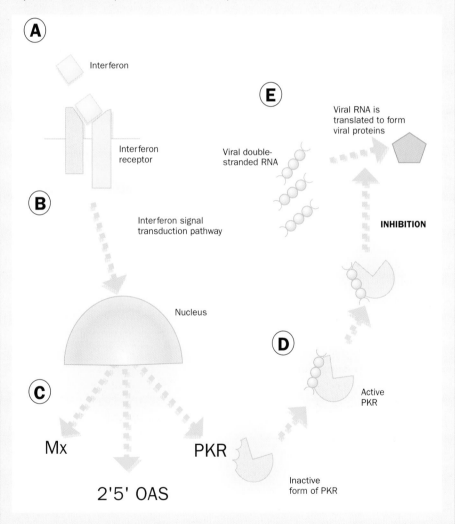

functions and the role they play in determining the outcome of the disease and the response to therapy is by no means clear and attempts to correlate the response to therapy with the sequence of the HCV-encoded interferon inhibitors have, to date, been unsuccessful. It now seems unlikely that sequencing of the HCV virus will allow prediction of the response to therapy in the foreseeable future.

Avoiding the acquired immune system

The acquired immune system provides long-lasting, pathogen-specific immunity and involves the production of antibodies and the generation of antiviral T cells. Circulating antibodies can neutralize virions, and they can bind to viral proteins that are expressed on the surface of cells and, by fixing complement, lyse them. Different classes of antibody are typically produced during different stages of an infection – initially IgM-type antibodies are produced but later IgG-type antibodies predominate. The identification of the type of circulating antibody may help distinguish acute from chronic infection.

Antiviral T cells are activated T lymphocytes that inhibit viral replication. Two groups of T lymphocytes may act as antiviral T cells: CD4-positive 'helper' T cells and CD8-positive 'cytotoxic' T cells. The CD4-positive T cells that inhibit viral replication belong to the Th1 group of CD4-positive T cells, and they inhibit viral replication by local production of antiviral cytokines (such as interferon gamma). The cytotoxic T cells (CD8-positive T cells) inhibit viral replication by lysing virally infected cells, either by producing lytic proteins or by activating endogenous apoptotic pathways by Fas/FasL interactions. For both of these antiviral T cells, close contact with the virally infected cell is essential for activity, and the activated T cells recognize virally infected cells only when the infected cells express viral antigens on their surface in association with HLA class I antigens. Surface expression of viral proteins by HLA class I antigens involves:

- cleavage of viral proteins by a collection of cellular enzymes (the proteosome);
- transport of the peptides into the endoplasmic reticulum by transporter (TAP) proteins; and
- cell surface presentation in association with HLA class I antigens.

The development and activation of antiviral lymphocytes is a complex process that involves:

- uptake of viral antigens by dendritic cells;
- presentation of viral peptides to helper T cells; and
- interaction between helper T cells and effector T cells, which leads to the generation of antiviral T cells.

The activated antiviral T cells recognize virally infected cells when the target cell expresses viral antigens in the context of HLA class I antigens on their surface. This presentation of viral antigens to T cells is enhanced by type I interferons, which upregulate HLA class I antigens (see page 3). The development of a cellular antiviral immune response is illustrated in Figure 1.2.

Figure 1.2

Generation of cellular immune responses. (A) Viral proteins from infected hepatocytes are ingested by dendritic cells (or the hepatocytes are themselves phagocytosed). The immature dendritic cells process the viral proteins (B) and migrate to the local lymph nodes, where they mature into 'professional' antigen-presenting cells (C). The mature antigen-presenting cells present the processed antigens on their surface in association with HLA class II antigens. Circulating T cells that recognize the foreign antigens activate (license) the antigen-presenting cells (D) and the activated antigen-presenting cells then interact with other lymphocytes (including cytotoxic T cells – CD8+ cells) and activate them (E). The activated T cells (both helper T cells (CD4+ T cells) and cytotoxic (CD8+ T cells)) migrate to the liver, where they identify infected cells that express foreign antigens on their surface in association with HLA class I antigens. The activated lymphocytes either inhibit viral replication, via local production of cytokines (Th1 cells) or induce lysis of the infected cells (CD8+ cells).

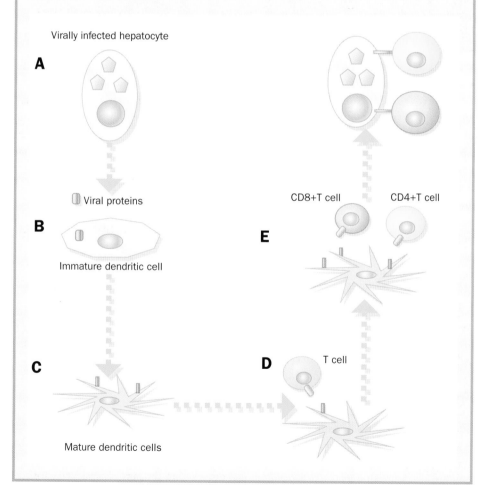

The development of an effective antiviral cellular immune response requires activation of the Th1 subset of helper T cells. Activation of the other helper T cell subset (Th2, CD4-positive T cells) inhibits activation of the Th1 cells and probably facilitates viral persistence. The factors that determine whether a Th1 or a Th2 T cell response develops are therefore critical in determining the outcome of a viral infection; at present, our understanding of these crucial control mechanisms remains incomplete and the details of how these different responses are controlled remain obscure.

Persistent viral infection is associated with avoidance of both arms of the immune system. The mechanisms of persistent viral infection are not completely understood but some general features are beginning to emerge. Mutation of viral proteins is a powerful avoidance strategy used by many viruses. Antibodies and circulating T cells recognize and bind to small, specific regions within viral proteins (epitopes). If these sequences change then the antibody or T cell can no longer recognize the viral protein and hence the virus can evade the antiviral defences. The hepatitis C virus uses this approach to avoid neutralizing antibodies – the envelope protein mutates at a high rate – and it is thought that cytotoxic T cells can be avoided by changes in other viral proteins. The hepatitis B virus avoids immune attacks based on the hepatitis B 'e' antigen (HBeAg) by mutating so that this protein is not produced at all (see page 69).

Viruses can also avoid the immune response by preventing activation of the system in the first instance. This effect can be specific or non-specific – the notorious human immunodeficiency virus (HIV) inhibits all immune responses by killing T cells, but the hepatotropic viruses are much more subtle and influence the immune system in multiple, albeit ill-understood, ways. The hepatitis B virus produces a small protein (HBeAg), which crosses the placenta and induces tolerance to itself, and related hepatitis B proteins. Because the immune system has come into contact with the protein in early life, the immune system believes the protein to be 'self' and is therefore unable to mount an effective immune response. The hepatitis C virus can also inhibit the generation of an appropriate immune response, and infection of dendritic cells is one mechanism that it appears to use to impair the development of a satisfactory immune response.

Prevalence, transmission and prevention of hepatitis

> Throughout the world, chronic infection with hepatotropic viruses is very common and over 500 million people are infected

Hepatitis C

Prevalence

The prevalence of hepatitis C virus infection varies between different countries, different regions and different population groups within the same country may have markedly different prevalence rates (Table 1.2). For example, in some Italian villages the prevalence may be as high as 20% whereas the prevalence in other parts of Italy is no greater than 2%.

In Europe as a whole, the prevalence of chronic hepatitis C virus infection increases along a north–south axis, with the northern, Scandinavian countries having a low prevalence (less than 0.5%) and the southern, Mediterranean countries having a higher prevalence, approaching 2%. The reasons for this variation are unclear.

The prevalence of chronic hepatitis C virus infection in the USA is similar to that in southern Europe (1.8%).

The prevalence in Africa is probably a little higher and is estimated to be around 2–5%.

In the Middle East, infection is common and affects between 1 and 12% of the population. The prevalence is particularly high in Egypt, where infection rates as high as 20% have been found. This unusually high prevalence is believed to be due to the use of unsterilized needles during therapy for schistosomiasis. The schistosomiasis eradication campaign may account for the high prevalence of hepatitis C virus infection in elderly Egyptians but, sadly, infection is also common in younger Egyptians – prevalence rates of as high as 10% have been seen in youngsters in Cairo who have not received therapy for schistosomiasis, and the high prevalence of hepatitis C virus infection in these individuals remains unexplained.

Transmission

> *Hepatitis C is a blood-borne virus that is transmitted through blood-to-blood contact – the virus is relatively difficult to pass on through casual contact and only those who have been in contact with infected blood are at high risk of infection*

Table 1.2
Prevalence of chronic hepatitis C infection in selected areas. Note that widespread epidemiological studies have not yet been performed, and the true prevalence and distribution of this virus have not yet been elucidated.

Continent	Country	Prevalence (%)	Comments
Europe	Sweden	0.3	Typical prevalence seen in northern Europe
	Italy (general)	2	
	Italy (Bari province)	26	Unusual cluster of cases
	Sardinia	7	
	Spain	0.8	
North America	USA	1.8	Based on a large, community survey
Africa	Cameroon	6.8	
	Egypt	26.6	

Because of the mode of transmission of hepatitis C virus, infection is common in those who have used intravenous drugs and in those who have shared injecting paraphernalia; it is also found in people who have received contaminated blood or blood products. In the developed world, transmission via blood products was curtailed in the early 1990s, when screening of all donated blood for hepatitis C began, and this route of transmission is now exceedingly rare.

Intravenous drug use carries the highest risk but nasal ingestion of cocaine (by snorting) may also transmit the virus, probably via blood-stained straws or other equipment. In addition to the common routes of transmission, a number of other modes of infection exist. Maternal–fetal transmission is rare and occurs in less than 5% of deliveries from mothers who are infected with hepatitis C. The risk of maternal–fetal transmission is increased if the mother has a high level of viraemia, and this is common in patients who are immunosuppressed. Hence maternal–fetal transmission is much more common in patients who are infected with both hepatitis C and HIV. Sexual transmission of hepatitis C is uncommon, although not impossible, and the prevalence of chronic hepatitis C virus infection in promiscuous people is only slightly greater than in those with few sexual partners. Percutaneous exposure with unsterilized piercing equipment (e.g. during body piercing or tattooing) may transmit the virus but this is now uncommon. Risk factors for chronic hepatitis C virus infection are shown in Table 1.3.

Medical staff may be infected with the hepatitis C virus via needle stick injuries from infected patients. This is extremely rare and recipients of needle stick injuries should be reassured that infection is unlikely. To confirm that infection has not occurred, a sample of the recipient's blood should be examined for the presence of the virus after 4 and 8 weeks (hepatitis C virus polymerase chain reaction test), and the absence of infection should be confirmed after 6 months by serological assays (hepatitis C virus antibody tests). It is also wise to perform a baseline test immediately after exposure to look for antibodies against hepatitis C to confirm that the person is not already infected. Early identification of individuals recently infected with hepatitis C virus is important as therapy, with interferon alone, in those who have acquired the infection within the last 6 months is very successful with viral eradication rates greater than 80%. Whether it is necessary to treat all acute hepatitis C infections or whether it is wiser to wait a few months to determine whether spontaneous clearance will occur is not yet clear and is the subject of ongoing clinical trials. The authors' current practice is to offer all patients with acute hepatitis C infection treatment but this advice may change as more data becomes available.

Infection of patients by infected healthcare personnel is extremely uncommon, but a few incidents of transmission have occurred in which an infected surgeon has infected a patient during an operation. Whether all surgeons should be screened for hepatitis C and barred from invasive procedures if found to be positive is a sensitive issue that is currently under consideration. Screening all

Table 1.3
Risk factors for infection with the hepatitis C virus.

Risk factor	Comments
Intravenous drug use	Most common mode of transmission in the developed world. The period of drug use may have ended many years before presentation
Other drug use (e.g. snorting cocaine)	Rare mode of transmission
Blood or blood product transfusion	Common in those transfused before 1990, but now very rare in developed countries
Incarceration	Infection is common in prisoners, probably as a result of drug abuse leading to incarceration or drug abuse in prison
Hospital therapy	Very rare mode of acquisition in the developed world. Remains a common route of transmission in many underdeveloped countries. Some medical procedures (e.g. dialysis) carry a very high risk and stringent precautions are required to prevent transmission
Infected mother	Risk is less than 5% unless the parent is also infected with HIV
Infected family member	Very low risk. Family members should not share blood-stained devices such as razors and toothbrushes
Body piercing	Very small risk
Promiscuity	Very low risk

surgeons and preventing those who are infected with hepatitis C from operating would prevent a very small number of transmissions, but the costs and the problems associated with reducing the number of operating surgeons would be considerable and many feel that the disadvantages outweigh the benefits.

Prevention

At present there is no effective vaccine against hepatitis C virus, and prevention of infection therefore relies on:

- screening of blood products for the virus; and

- prevention of transmission among active drug users by appropriate education and provision of clean injecting paraphernalia.

It is important to recognize that intravenous drug users may transmit the virus by contact with contaminated injecting paraphernalia (such as tourniquets, spoons etc – known colloquially as 'the works'), and therefore simple provision of clean needles and advice not to share needles may not be sufficient to prevent the spread of hepatitis C. Injecting drug users must be advised not to share any item of injecting equipment.

Hepatitis B

Prevalence

Hepatitis B virus is an extremely common virus throughout the world. It is endemic in many populations, ranging from the Inuit in Alaska to the Polynesian islanders in the south Pacific. In endemic parts of the world – Africa, the Far East and the Amazon basin – up to 80% of the population have evidence of exposure to hepatitis B virus and up to 20% are actively infected. In the developed world hepatitis B is uncommon and the prevalence varies from 5 to 10% in the Mediterranean countries to less than 2% in northern Europe and the USA. The prevalence of hepatitis B virus infection around the world is shown in Figure 1.3.

Transmission

The hepatitis B virus is extremely infectious and is readily transmitted by blood-to-blood contact. An interesting, but unexplained, observation is that in Asia transmission occurs from mothers to their infants during childbirth, but in Africa the virus is passed on in early childhood. Many of these infected children go on to eliminate the virus and the persistence of viral antibodies is the only evidence of exposure; however, others go on to become chronically infected.

In areas of the world where hepatitis B is not endemic, the virus is easily transmitted to non-vaccinated people by close contact with those who are infected. In contrast with hepatitis C, the hepatitis B virus is very infectious and exposure to miniscule

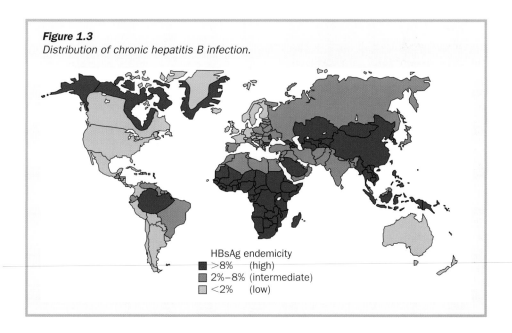

Figure 1.3
Distribution of chronic hepatitis B infection.

HBsAg endemicity
- >8% (high)
- 2%–8% (intermediate)
- <2% (low)

amounts of blood is sufficient to transmit the pathogen.

Sexual transmission occurs, and hepatitis B virus is more often found in those who are promiscuous, particularly in men who have sex with men. The virus may be passed on by drug misuse but in many Western countries the virus has not become established in the drug-using community and hence relatively few intravenous drug users are infected. Over the past few years the increase in young adults travelling to exotic holiday locations has led to an increase in hepatitis B virus infection in this group and teenagers with hepatitis B virus infection should be questioned carefully about recent sexual experiences abroad.

Healthcare workers who are infected with hepatitis B virus may transmit the virus to patients during invasive procedures. Those who are most likely to transmit the virus are:

- those who are HBeAg-positive; and
- those who are HBeAg-negative but have high levels of circulating virus.

In many countries such healthcare workers are barred from performing exposure-prone invasive procedures. (The definition of 'high levels of circulating virus' differs from country to country. Some authorities consider 'high level' to be more than 10^5 copies/ml, whereas others regard 3×10^4 copies/ml (the lowest level at which transmission has been documented) as 'high level'.)

Prevention

The surface antigen of hepatitis B is highly immunogenic and causes prolonged immunity in the majority of vaccinated people. The original hepatitis B vaccines were derived from the serum of patients who had partially eliminated the virus, but the current vaccines are derived from genetically engineered yeast; hence there is no risk of infection with other blood-borne pathogens during vaccination. Following vaccination antibodies against HBsAg (anti-HBs) develop and a circulating antibody titre of more than 1 in 100 is regarded as protective. If the titre falls to approaching this level a booster vaccination should be considered. A few individuals do not respond to the current vaccine, and for these individuals active vaccination is not possible at present. If unprotected individuals (either unvaccinated or vaccine non-responders) are inadvertently exposed to hepatitis B virus the early (within 24 hours) intramuscular administration of hepatitis B immunoglobulin (HBIg) at a dose of 500 IU may prevent transmission. In those who have not been previously vaccinated this passive protection should be followed by a full course of vaccination to provide long-term protection.

There is ongoing debate as to whether all hepatitis B vaccine recipients should be tested for the presence of antibodies and offered booster vaccinations at regular intervals. The current consensus is that such an approach is unnecessary (the anamnestic response to the first vaccination schedule should provide sufficient protection against further exposure), but in people at very high risk (e.g. medical personnel) it may be prudent to adopt a more cautious approach and maintain high titres of protective antibody, as outlined above. The introduction of global vaccination in parts of the world where hepatitis B virus infection is common (e.g. Italy and Taiwan) has led to a fall in the prevalence of hepatocellular carcinoma, indicating that vaccination is an effective means of reducing the mortality and morbidity of chronic hepatitis B virus infection.

Hepatitis delta

Infection with the delta virus is possible only in people who are also infected with hepatitis B virus. The delta virus may be contracted either simultaneously with the hepatitis B virus (co-infection) or later (superinfection). Hence the virus is common only in areas where hepatitis B is endemic. However, not all areas that have a high prevalence of hepatitis B have a high rate of hepatitis delta superinfection. For example, the virus is rare in most of southern Africa but common in Venezuela and some Mediterranean countries.

The delta virus is a blood-borne virus that may be transmitted by parenteral contact. In developed countries, the virus is normally associated with intravenous drug use although in some countries (in particular Romania) nosocomial transmission from contaminated medical equipment has led to high prevalence in some populations. In South America, epidemics of the virus with high mortality occur infrequently, but the route of transmission in these outbreaks is not yet clear. Sexual transmission of the delta virus is uncommon.

Prevention of infection with the delta virus relies on effective prevention of hepatitis B virus infection by vaccination.

Other hepatotropic viruses

A small number of patients develop chronic hepatitis that appears to be transmitted by blood or blood products but is not due to one of the currently identified hepatitis viruses – this is known as non-A–E hepatitis. The virus responsible for this infection has not been identified but a number of possible aetiological agents have been proposed. These include hepatitis G virus (also known as GBV-C) and the transfusion transmitted virus (TTV). A number of epidemiological studies have shown that these agents are unlikely to be the cause of most cases of non-A–E hepatitis, and it is likely that these viruses do not cause significant liver disease.

Further reading

Basic science

Racanelli V, Rehermann B. Hepatitis C virus infection: when silence is deception. *Trends Immunol* 2003; **24**: 456–64.

Ferrari C, Missale G, Boni C, Urbani S. Immunopathogenesis of hepatitis B. *J Hepatol* 2003; **39**: S36–42.

Pestka S, Langer T, Zoon K, Samuel C. Interferons and their actions. *Annu Rev Biochem* 1987; **56**: 727–77.

Epidemiology

Lavanchy D. Hepatitis B virus epidemiology, disease burden treatment and current and emerging prevention and control measures. *J Viral Hepat* 2004; **11**: 97–107.

World Health Organization. Global surveillance and control of hepatitis C. *J Viral Hepat* 1999; **6**: 35–47.

Questions

1. Regarding chronic hepatitis B virus
    infection in Africa:
    A. Over 80% of the population are
        actively infected
    B. Maternal–fetal transmission usually
        occurs in utero
    C. Sexual transmission does not occur
    D. Chronic infection has a good
        prognosis
    E. Co-infection with hepatitis C is
        common

2. Regarding chronic hepatitis C virus
    infection:
    A. It is common in prostitutes who do
        not use drugs
    B. Transmission between intravenous
        drug users can be eliminated by
        needle exchange programmes
    C. It is rarely passed from mothers to
        their children
    D. It may be passed on from infected
        healthcare personnel
    E. Transmission can be prevented by
        vaccination

3. Infection with the delta virus:
    A. Can be prevented by successful
        vaccination against hepatitis B virus
    B. Is always associated with chronic
        hepatitis C virus infection
    C. Never causes severe disease
    D. Is common in northern Europe
    E. May cause outbreaks of hepatitis

4. The type I interferons:
    A. Inhibit the replication of the
        hepatitis B virus by the effects of the
        protein kinase PKR
    B. Are induced within a few hours of
        viral infection
    C. May be inhibited by viral infection
    D. Are of little importance in
        eliminating viral infections
    E. Enhance immune recognition of
        virally infected cells

Answers

Question 1

A. False – active infection with viraemia affects no more than 20% of the population
B. False – maternal–fetal transmission occurs during delivery or early life
C. False
D. False
E. False

Question 2

A. False – sexual transmission is rare and infection in sex workers is unusual unless they also abuse drugs
B. False – the virus can be transmitted on injecting paraphernalia
C. True
D. True
E. False

Question 3

A. True
B. False – it is associated with hepatitis B virus infection
C. False – it typically causes more severe disease
D. False
E. True

Question 4

A. False – it is not yet clear how interferon inhibits the replication of hepatitis B virus, but PKR, which is active against double-stranded RNA viruses, is unlikely to be involved
B. True
C. True
D. False – they are crucial, and genetically engineered mice that do not respond to interferon die rapidly from normally trivial viral infections
E. True

Hepatitis C – virology, natural history and pathology

2

Since its discovery in 1989 the hepatitis C virus has been extensively studied by both academic and commercial research groups. However, progress has been relatively slow and our current knowledge remains fragmentary. The natural history of the disease caused by the hepatitis C virus (formally known as non-A non-B hepatitis) has proved difficult to study because there is no appropriate small animal model. Hence, much of our present understanding about this virus and its associated disease is likely to change over the next few years.

Hepatitis C – the virus

The hepatitis C virus has been visualized by electron microscopy as an enveloped virus-like particle, 50–60 nm in diameter. To date there is no *in vitro* replication system that allows a full analysis of the viral replication cycle. However, the development of models of intracellular replication based upon self-replicating hepatitis C-derived RNAs (the HCV replicon) has allowed studies of the replication of HCV RNA that have greatly increased our understanding of this virus.

Viral structure

The hepatitis C virus genome consists of a single strand of RNA that is directly processed to produce the viral proteins (i.e. it is a positive-strand RNA virus). The genome is very similar to viruses in the Flaviviridae family (such as the yellow fever and dengue viruses) and, by analogy, the functions of the different regions of the hepatitis C virus genome have been identified. These are shown in Figure 2.1.

In common with many RNA viruses, the hepatitis C virus mutates at a very high rate. This means that in any infected patient there are multiple different viruses, each differing by a few nucleotides, and one or two amino acids – in other words, the virus exists as a population of closely related but different viral species (quasispecies). Over time some of these different viral species are more successful and become dominant, so that the viral population changes. It is estimated that the dominant viral sequence changes every few weeks. These changes may help the hepatitis C virus to avoid the immune system. Since the genomic sequence of the hepatitis C virus changes every few weeks it is not surprising to find that every patient is infected with a slightly different 'viral cocktail' and no two people will have an identical viral population. However, people who are initially infected with the same virus will develop a viral population that is related, and by examining the sequence of the viruses one can examine the possibility that two people were infected from a common source. These types of analysis are of obvious value in investigating iatrogenic and other outbreaks.

Within the hepatitis C virus there are regions that are reasonably stable and change relatively little (these include the non-coding regions and the hepatitis C virus core protein). The slow evolution of these conserved regions has differed in different geographical regions and has led to the evolution of different strains of hepatitis C virus, known as genotypes.

At least six genotypes are now recognized (Table 2.1). All of the different genotypes appear to have a similar effect on

---

Figure 2.1

Schematic representation of the proteins encoded by the hepatitis C virus genome. The genome consists of a non-coding region, the 5' untranslated region (UTR) linked to a coding region that encodes the proteins illustrated in the figure. At the 5' end of the virus the RNA encodes the structural proteins (core (C) and the envelope proteins E1 and E2). The function of the small p7 protein is unknown. Following the structural proteins are the non-structural proteins (the NS proteins). NS2 is a protease that cleaves the viral polyprotein, NS3 is a complex protein that encodes a helicase and a protease and NS4A is a co-factor that binds to and activates NS3. NS5 is split into two proteins – NS5A is of unknown function but may inhibit the cellular response to interferon and NS5B is an RNA polymerase that replicates the viral genome.

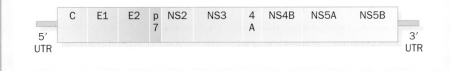

Table 2.1
Genotypes of the hepatitis C virus and their main characteristics.

Genotype	Distribution	Response to interferon and ribavirin therapy	Comments
1	Worldwide	Modest (40–50%) – 48 weeks of therapy are required	Most common genotype in Europe, USA and Japan
2	Worldwide	Good (70–80%) – 24 weeks of therapy required	
3	Worldwide	Good (70–80%)– 24 weeks of therapy required	Common in drug users in the developed world
4	Middle East	Good (60–80%) – 48 weeks of therapy are probably required, but few data are available	
5	Far East	Unknown	
6	South Africa	Unknown	

the liver (i.e. disease progression is similar for all of them) but the response to therapy is strongly influenced by genotype, and different durations of treatment are required to treat the different genotypes (see page 48). These genotypes can be subdivided (e.g. genotype 1 has been subdivided into type 1a and type 1b) but this is not of value in clinical practice.

Replication of the hepatitis C virus

Our knowledge of the replication of the hepatitis C virus is still incomplete and details of viral entry and exit from cells is particularily scanty. The information that is currently available is being used to develop new antiviral agents and it is likely that the currently identified drug targets will lead to novel therapeutic agents in the foreseeable future.

The hepatitis C virus enters a hepatocyte by binding to a specific cell surface receptor. The receptor has not yet been clearly identified although the cell surface protein CD81 is an HCV-binding protein that may play a role in viral entry. The regions within the envelope protein that interact with the receptor have not been identified, but they are probably encoded by the E1 protein or the E2 protein, or possibly both. A complete understanding of the interaction between the hepatitis C virus and its receptor will allow predictions of crucial, invariate regions of the envelope protein. This will greatly facilitate vaccine designs, since vaccines targeted against these regions are unlikely to allow for the development of vaccine escape mutants.

Following entry into the cell the hepatitis C genome is translated by host ribosomes to produce a single large protein, the polyprotein. The 5′ untranslated region of the hepatitis C virus plays a key role in this process and, since this region is highly conserved between different viral isolates, it may be possible to develop drugs that bind to this region and inhibit viral translation. The polyprotein that is produced by translation of the hepatitis C virus genome is cleaved and processed to form a replication complex that associates with the endoplasmic reticulum. Cleavage of the hepatitis C polyprotein involves a number of proteases, including the non-structural (NS) proteins of the virus, NS2 and the NS3–4. The viral proteases from other viruses have been successfully inhibited by compounds that are therapeutically valuable, and hence the protease of hepatitis C is an attractive target for drug development. Early clinical studies with HCV NS3 protease inhibitors have been reported and shown to effectively inhibit viral replication in the short term. However, the long-term safety and efficacy of these prototypes have not yet been evaluated. It is probable that effective drugs that target the protease will be tested in patients over the next few years and results from these trials are awaited with great interest.

Cleavage of the viral polyprotein releases and activates other viral proteins. The key proteins involved in the replication of the viral genome are the helicase protein (encoded by the NS3 region) and the polymerase protein (encoded by the NS5B region). These two proteins are required for the production of new hepatitis C viral RNA strands and thus are attractive targets for novel antiviral agents and preliminary reports show that inhibitors of the HCV

polymerase do inhibit viral replication in humans. Again, long-term studies are required to assess the value of these novel agents and it is likely that polymerase inhibitors will enter clinical trials in the foreseeable future. The newly formed viral RNA strands are packaged into novel viral particles and released by mechanisms that are, as yet, poorly understood. The bovine diarrhoea virus, which is a closely related virus, is released from cells only after extensive glycosylation, and inhibiting this process inhibits the release of the virus. Since the envelope proteins of the hepatitis C virus are also glycosylated, it is possible that drugs that inhibit glycosylation may have activity against hepatitis C virus – this approach is under investigation.

Natural history of hepatitis C virus infection

Infection with the hepatitis C virus occasionally causes acute hepatitis, in which the patient becomes overtly jaundiced with markedly raised serum transaminases. However, most patients are unknowingly infected and are asymptomatic at the time of infection. Chronic infection with the hepatitis C virus leads to a disease whose outcome is extremely variable.

A small proportion (estimated to be around 20–50%) of patients clear the virus and remain persistently non-viraemic with normal liver function tests. Exposure to the virus in these patients can be inferred from the presence of antibodies against the virus in the absence of detectable viraemia although some studies have shown that the antibodies against hepatitis C virus can disappear with time leaving no clear evidence of infection. Recurrence of viraemia in such patients has not been reported and is unlikely, although profound immunosuppression might, in theory, lead to reactivation.

For the 50–80% of exposed patients who develop a persistent infection spontaneous clearance is rare, and patients who are hepatitis C viraemic 12 months after exposure are very unlikely to clear the virus without therapy.

Some patients are infected with the hepatitis C virus for decades and, after 20–30 years, a liver biopsy shows minimal disease with no scarring. However, in others the disease progresses much more rapidly and within 10 years the liver inflammation and fibrosis lead to cirrhosis. In the majority of patients, the virus causes a slowly progressive fibrosis that leads to cirrhosis in more than three decades.

It is assumed by some that the progression of fibrosis in chronic hepatitis C is linear and that the fibrosis slowly increases with time. This may not always be the case and in some patients quiescent disease may become active and the fibrosis may progress very rapidly. In others active disease with rapid scarring may slow, and some believe that the scarring may even reverse. Certainly fibrosis may be reversible following treatment. Figure 2.2 illustrates the natural history of chronic hepatitis C virus infection.

In most patients with chronic infection the liver function tests fluctuate and may vary from normal to markedly raised over the space of a few days. Hence the traditional 'liver function tests' – serum transaminases, alkaline phosphatase

bilirubin and albumin are very poor predictors of liver damage in patients with chronic hepatitis C virus and the only reliable way to assess this disease is to perform a liver biopsy. New imaging and biochemical tests may help reduce the need for liver biopsy and these technologies are currently under evaluation. The available tests may be able to identify patients with mild or severe disease but are less reliable for identifying patients with disease of intermediate severity. The value of performing a liver biopsy, with its attendant risks and costs, in patients with hepatitis C virus genotypes which respond very well to therapy (genotypes 2 and 3) is questioned by many.

The factors that influence the progression of chronic hepatitis C virus infection are still largely unknown. Patients who are male and who contract the virus late in life (after the age of 40 years) tend to have more aggressive disease with more rapid development of the fibrosis. However, in an individual patient it is impossible to predict the rate of progression of the disease. Excessive alcohol consumption (more than 40 g/day) accelerates the disease in all patients and should be avoided. Most authorities agree that moderate alcohol consumption increases the rate of disease progression and is best avoided, but occasional consumption is probably of little consequence. Similarly, those patients with risk factors for non-alcoholic steatohepatitis (NASH) are more likely to have progressive disease. Co-existing haemochromatosis or HIV infection are also associated with an increase in the rate of disease progression.

For patients with hepatitis C-related cirrhosis, the outlook is bleak. Every year a

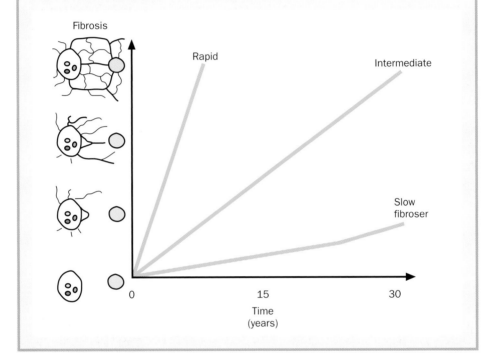

Figure 2.2
Fibrosis is shown by the METAVIR scoring system and time is shown in years. In some patients the fibrosis progresses rapidly such that cirrhosis is present within 10 years. In contrast other patients do not develop any significant fibrosis within 30 years. The majority of patients progress very slowly such that 30% have cirrhosis after 30 years.

small percentage (around 3–5%) of such patients develop liver cell cancer and 1–3% develop decompensated liver disease. Without successful therapy or transplantation, death from cirrhosis and its complications is inevitable.

Pathology of hepatitis C

Histopathological features of chronic hepatitis C virus infection

A number of histopathological features have been described as being characteristic of

hepatitis C virus infection (Table 2.2). The three most common of these are:

- the presence of portal lymphoid follicles and aggregates (Figure 2.3);
- 'hepatitic' bile duct damage (Figure 2.4); and
- fatty change (Figure 2.5).

Lymphoid aggregates may be seen in other causes of chronic hepatitis, such as autoimmune hepatitis and even some cases of hepatitis B. Nevertheless they are much more common in hepatitis C, in which

Figure 2.3
Liver biopsy from a case of chronic HCV with a characteristic portal tract lymphoid aggregate. There is no piecemeal necrosis/interface hepatitis.

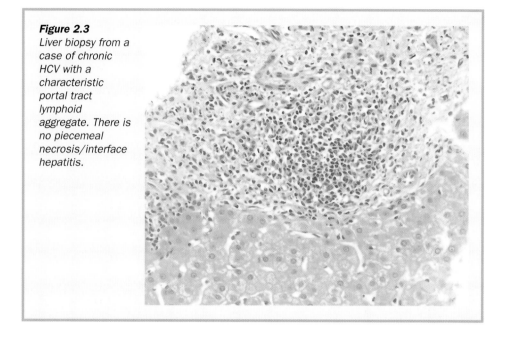

Figure 2.4
Liver biopsy from a case of chronic HCV with characteristic bile duct damage (but not bile duct loss).

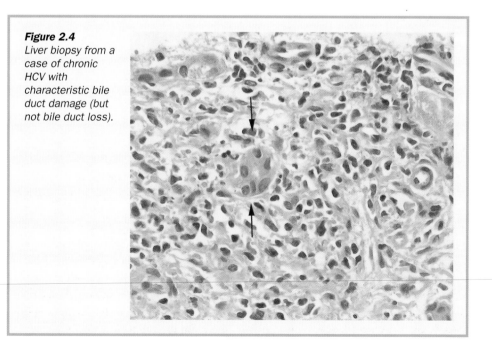

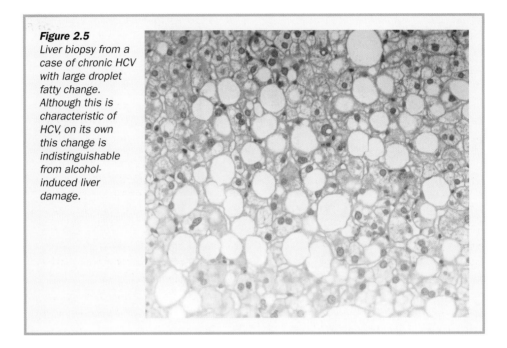

Figure 2.5
Liver biopsy from a case of chronic HCV with large droplet fatty change. Although this is characteristic of HCV, on its own this change is indistinguishable from alcohol-induced liver damage.

Table 2.2

Characteristic histological features of chronic hepatitis C.

Portal lymphoid follicles and aggregates
'Hepatitic' bile duct damage
Fatty change
Borderline interface hepatitis
Prominent lobular inflammation

they tend to be better formed. In some cases of hepatitis C, the lymphoid aggregates have well-formed germinal centres which contain follicle centre cells and dendritic cells. They are surrounded by a mantle zone that is rich in B cells, which is in turn surrounded by a zone that is rich in CD4-positive T cells. Well-formed lymphoid follicles are most often seen in

cases with otherwise relatively inactive disease. Their presence can be highlighted using a reticulin stain.

'Hepatitic' bile duct damage is also very common in hepatitis C virus infection. This damage is characterized by an inflammatory infiltrate that extends into the biliary epithelium, which itself shows degenerative changes, including cytoplasmic vacuolation and reactive nuclear changes (e.g. stratification and nuclear crowding). The key point is that there is no bile duct loss – bile duct loss in a patient with hepatitis C should initiate a search for another cause, such as primary sclerosing cholangitis. Canalicular cholestasis is also exceptionally uncommon in chronic hepatitis C virus infection, and its presence should prompt a search for an additional cause of liver disease – the most common are drug-induced hepatitis and superimposed acute viral hepatitis (most usually infection with hepatitis A virus).

Fatty change is common in hepatitis C virus infection, especially in patients infected with genotype 3, as it is in many liver diseases, including, of course, alcohol-induced liver disease and diabetes/obesity. A relatively common question asked of pathologists is whether the liver damage seen in a biopsy from a patient with hepatitis C who also drinks alcohol is due mainly to the infection or to the alcohol intake. The presence, distribution and severity of the fatty change is of no help in making this decision. The presence of significant alcohol-induced liver injury can only be made when the biopsy shows:

- ballooning degeneration of hepatocytes with Mallory's hyaline stain (Figure 2.6);
- a neutrophilic infiltrate (Figure 2.6); and
- pericellular fibrosis (Figure 2.7).

Neither Mallory's hyaline nor pericellular fibrosis are seen in cases of uncomplicated hepatitis C (despite claims to the contrary!). In rare cases, the presence of one or (more significantly) more of these three changes in a patient in whom hepatitis C virus infection is unsuspected should suggest the need for rechecking the serology. This is particularly true in acute hepatitis C in which the serology is not always reliable. It should be noted that in cases of acute hepatitis C virus infection these three characteristic histological features are often seen. In patients with co-existing hepatitis

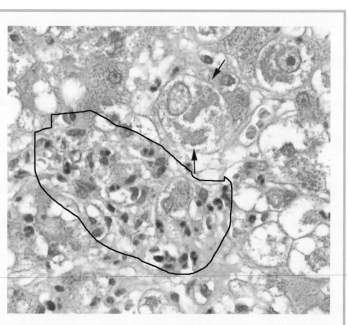

Figure 2.6
Liver biopsy from a patient with HCV who drinks excessively. The biopsy shows neutrophilic inflammation (within the enclosed area) and Mallory's hyaline within ballooned hepatocytes (one of which is arrowed). This indicates that alcohol is a significant contributing factor to this patient's liver damage.

Figure 2.7
Liver biopsy from
the same patient
as in Figure 2.6
showing pericellular
fibrosis which is
also characteristic
of alcohol induced
liver damage
(trichrome stain).

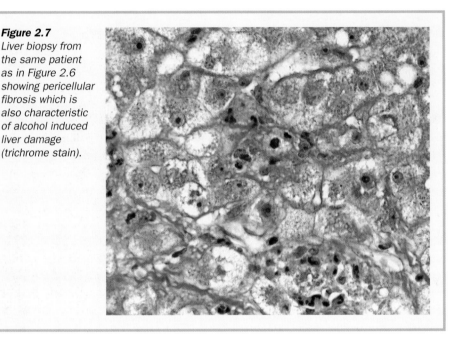

C and hepatitis B features of both diseases are seen.

It is typical of hepatitis C virus infection that the degree of interface hepatitis is usually mild and the degree of lobular inflammation is often greater than that seen in hepatitis B virus infection (Figures 2.8–2.11). This is one of the reasons why the classification of chronic hepatitis into chronic persistent hepatitis and chronic active hepatitis, which depends entirely on the presence or absence of interface hepatitis 'piecemeal necrosis', has fallen into disuse. Prominent acidophilic degeneration of hepatocytes that leads to the formation of apoptotic bodies is characteristic of hepatitis C. The lobular inflammation can take the form of a widespread sinusoidal infiltrate that is similar to the picture seen

with the Epstein–Barr virus. Granulomas are more common in chronic hepatitis C than in chronic hepatitis B. However, if a granuloma is seen in a patient with hepatitis C virus infection, every effort should be made to exclude other causes of hepatic granulomas (e.g. tuberculosis, sarcoidosis). Large or small cell hepatocyte dysplasia (change) may also be seen, especially in cirrhotic livers (see page 134).

Immunohistochemical staining has no role to play in the routine assessment of liver biopsies in patients with hepatitis C because no commercially available antibody has been shown to work reliably on formalin-fixed, paraffin-embedded tissue. *In situ* polymerase chain reaction (PCR) to detect the viral RNA in tissue is also not used in clinical practice. As is the case with

Figure 2.8
Liver biopsy from a patient with HCV showing apoptosis which is a common form of liver cell damage in this form of hepatitis. It is uncommon in HBV except when there is co-existent HDV.

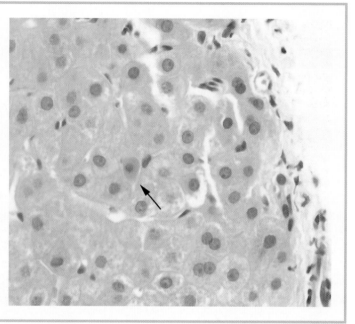

Figure 2.9
The same case as in Figure 2.8 with a sinusoidal pattern of lymphoid infiltration (arrowed) which is seen in HCV and also in infectious mononucleosis.

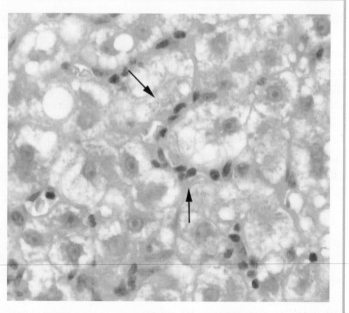

Figure 2.10
Liver biopsy from a patient with HCV with irregularity of the limiting plate (i.e. the interface between the connective tissue of the portal tract and the hepatocytes in the lobules) indicative of interface hepatitis (piecemeal necrosis).

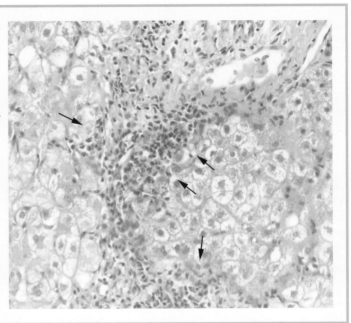

Figure 2.11
Liver biopsy from the same patient as in Figure 2.10 showing, at a higher power, a periportal hepatocyte (arrowed) surrounding by lymphocytes and which shows degenerative features. This is the defining feature of interface hepatitis (piecemeal necrosis).

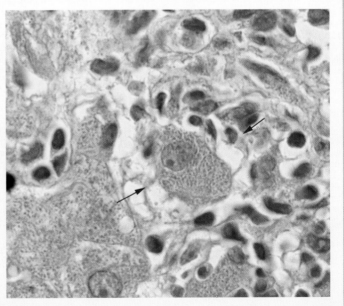

hepatitis B, PCR for the virus on liver tissue may be positive even if it has been negative in the serum. Given the frequency with which patients with hepatitis C undergo liver biopsy it is not surprising that some of them are also found to have another type of liver disease. The most common of these are:

- alcohol-induced liver disease; and
- genetic haemochromatosis.

The interpretation of alcohol-induced changes in patients with hepatitis C has been discussed above. To assess the degree of iron overload, and its distribution, it is necessary for all liver biopsies to be stained specifically for iron (Perls' Prussian blue reaction) (Figures 2.12 and 2.13). In genetic haemochromatosis iron is deposited in the hepatocytes. In cirrhotic livers, parenchymal iron may be seen in patients with no other evidence of genetic haemochromatosis. Nevertheless the presence of any iron in the hepatocytes raises the possibility of genetic haemochromatosis, which must be excluded by appropriate iron studies. This pattern needs to be distinguished from haemosiderosis, in which iron is deposited in the Kupffer cells. There are a number of causes for the latter appearance but in patients with hepatitis C the most common is treatment with ribavirin, which induces haemolytic anaemia, and blood transfusion. Particularly in Egyptian patients, schistosome eggs may be identified within the portal tracts.

Sometimes in patients with hepatitis C, the liver biopsy may also provide a clue as

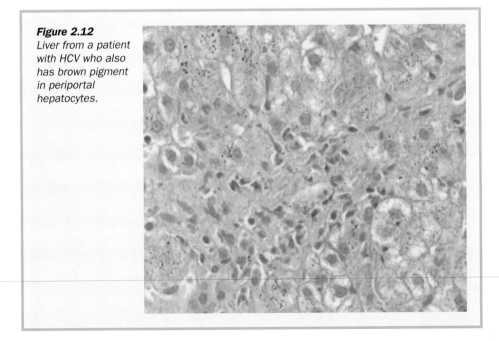

Figure 2.12
Liver from a patient with HCV who also has brown pigment in periportal hepatocytes.

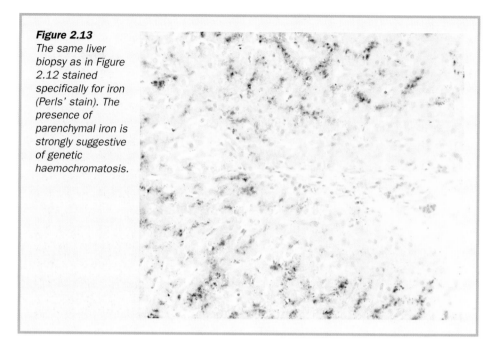

Figure 2.13
The same liver biopsy as in Figure 2.12 stained specifically for iron (Perls' stain). The presence of parenchymal iron is strongly suggestive of genetic haemochromatosis.

to the means whereby the hepatitis C virus was contracted. For example, the presence of refractile foreign material, including talc particles, in the portal tracts is typically seen in patients who are past or present intravenous drug users. Examining sections under polarized light is helpful in identifying these particles.

Grading and staging of chronic viral hepatitis

The grading and staging of chronic viral hepatitis, and especially hepatitis C, has become a common, albeit much debated, undertaking. One of the most important recent conceptual developments in liver pathology has been the realization that when assessing liver biopsies from patients

with chronic hepatitis it is essential to make a separate assessment of the severity of the necroinflammatory changes and the fibrotic changes. These two types of change are described by:

- the grade (for the necroinflammatory changes); and
- the stage (for fibrosis).

Grade essentially summarizes the overall severity of the inflammatory changes (Figures 2.8–2.11, 2.14) that are seen in and around the portal tracts and within the lobules, while stage provides information as to how far down the road to cirrhosis the patient has travelled (Figures 2.15–2.17). These terms were coined by analogy with the grading and staging of cancers. The grade depends on

Figure 2.14
Liver biopsy
showing a normal
portal tract with
scanty lymphocytes.

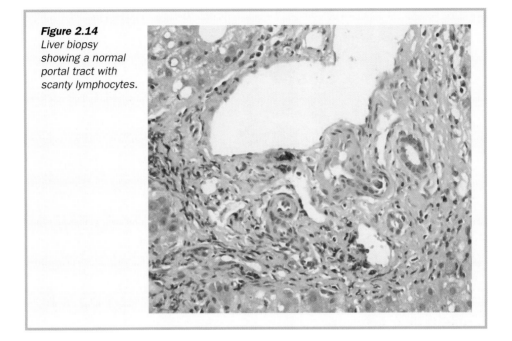

Figure 2.15
Liver biopsy
showing a normal
portal tract
(Reticulin stain). On
all of the scoring
systems described
this is Stage 0
disease.

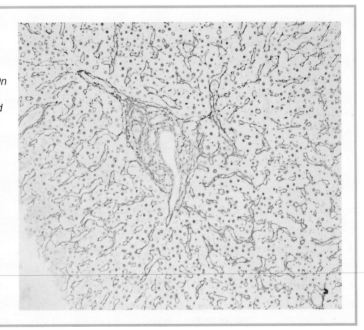

Figure 2.16
Liver biopsy
showing bridging
fibrosis with a
portal tract
connected to a
central vein by
connective tissue
(Reticulin stain).

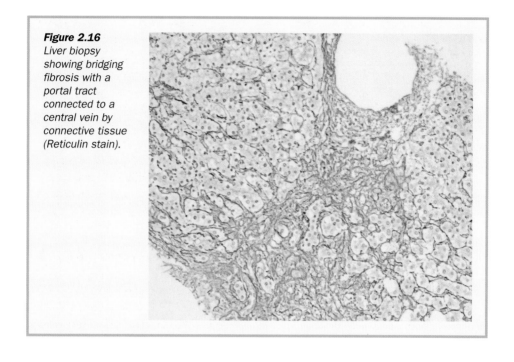

Figure 2.17
A cirrhotic liver with
nodules of
regenerating
hepatocytes
surrounded by cuffs
of fibrous tissue.

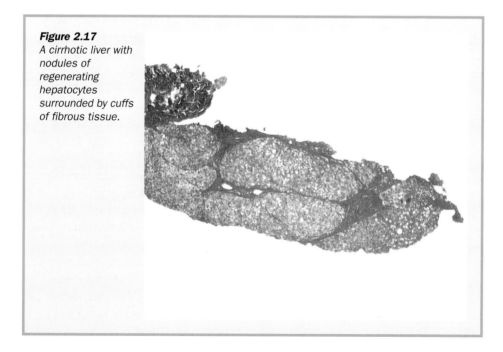

host and viral factors as well as on the effects of treatment, and it may wax and wane, especially in hepatitis C. On the other hand, until recently fibrosis (measured by stage) was thought to be an irreversible process (see page 121). It should, nevertheless, be made clear that inflammation and fibrosis are related to each other pathophysiologically.

While the definitions of portal and lobular inflammation are straightforward, the definition of interface hepatitis ('piecemeal necrosis') is less so. It is defined by two features:

- portal inflammation crossing the limiting plate (which is the line that separates the connective tissue of the portal tract from the hepatocytes) and extending into the lobules; and
- the presence of degenerative changes in the periportal hepatocytes.

The second feature distinguishes interface hepatitis from simple 'spill-over' of portal tract inflammation into the lobules, although in practice this distinction is very difficult. The term 'piecemeal necrosis' was coined to describe this progressive nibbling away of hepatocytes adjacent to the limiting plate. Purists object to this term because the mode of cell death seen is in fact apoptosis and not necrosis. For this reason the terms 'interface hepatitis' or 'periportal inflammation' have been suggested as being more accurate terms and the former is used here. However, as is so often the case when it comes to medical terminology, the use of the older term is likely to continue for some time to come! It is important to note that interface hepatitis can be seen not only

in chronic hepatitis, of any cause, but also in other diseases such as primary biliary cirrhosis and Wilson's disease.

A number of different semiquantitative scoring systems have been proposed for assessing the grade and stage of the histopathological changes seen in chronic hepatitis C. These can be (and have been) applied to other causes of chronic hepatitis but have been studied in most detail with reference to hepatitis C and are therefore discussed here. The four most widely used systems (Table 2.3) are:

- the histological activity index (HAI) or Knodell scoring system;
- the Scheuer scoring system;
- the METAVIR scoring system; and
- the modified HAI (Ishak) scoring system.

The Knodell (HAI) scoring system

The Knodell scoring system is the oldest liver biopsy scoring system. In its original form the scores for portal, periportal and lobular inflammation were added to the fibrosis score to give an overall HAI. After the importance of separating the necroinflammatory (grade) and fibrosis (stage) scores was appreciated (see page 30), this system has been modified. The scores for the inflammatory components have been split off; when added together they give the Knodell HAI inflammation score. The fibrosis gives the Knodell HAI fibrosis score.

An idiosyncrasy of the Knodell scoring system is that the scores for the individual components are 0, 1, 3 and 4 (i.e. there is no 2). The reason for this is not clear but it does have the effect of separating scores into low-score (0 and 1) and high-score

Table 2.3
Summary of the four main biopsy scoring systems for chronic hepatitis.

Scoring system	Maximum stage score	Maximum grade score	Comments
HAI (Knodell)	4	18	The original scoring system, which has been modified to separate stage and grade
Scheuer	4	4	The first scoring system to separate stage and grade
METAVIR	4	4	An excellent scoring system
Modified HAI (Ishak)	6	18	The most widely used scoring system in the UK and the USA

groups (3 and 4) with no intermediate groups. This feature is, however, an ongoing source of frustration to statisticians analysing studies in which this scoring system has been used.

Despite this drawback, the Knodell scoring system remains the one most widely used in clinical trials. It is a robust system that has been used for some time.

The Scheuer scoring system

Although not widely used except in Australia, the importance of the classical paper in which the Scheuer scoring system was described is that it was the first paper in which the importance of separating inflammatory and fibrosis scores was clearly stated and the first paper to use the terms 'grade' and 'stage' in this context.

The METAVIR scoring system

The METAVIR scoring system is an excellent scoring system that was developed by a group of French pathologists. It is the best validated of all the scoring systems in terms of its reproducibility and clinical application. The overall necroinflammatory score is read off a grid that has the score for interface hepatitis along one axis and the score for lobular inflammation along the other. The degree of portal inflammation is ignored because it is considered to be less important than interface hepatitis and lobular inflammation in producing liver damage. Unfortunately this system has not been widely used outside France.

The Ishak (modified HAI) scoring system

The Ishak scoring system (Table 2.4) is essentially an update of the Knodell (HAI) scoring system – grade and stage are clearly separated and there is no missing number in the scores for each feature (e.g. the scores for fibrosis are 0, 1, 2, 3, 4, 5, 6). In addition, there is a separate scoring category for confluent necrosis. It should be noted that confluent necrosis is in fact very unusual in chronic hepatitis C virus infection. Another modification is that there are more points on each scale. For example, in the Knodell scoring system, there are four possible scores for fibrosis whereas in the Ishak scoring system there are seven. Although this increased sensitivity may appear an advantage it is not clear if this feature is of benefit either in clinical practice or in trials. The reproducibility of this scoring system has been shown to be less than for the three other main scoring systems.

Overall comments

All the scoring systems described above have much in common. In all of them the scores for the individual histological features are ordinal data – that is, the scores increase with increasing severity of pathology – but the differences between the individual scores are not equal (and in fact are not known). For example, in the Ishak scoring system 0 means no fibrosis, 1 means focal portal tract expansion, while 2 means generalized portal tract expansion and 3 means focal bridging fibrosis. However, the significance of a change of a score from 0 to 1 is unlikely to be the same as the significance of a score from 2 to 3 – the latter change is likely to be more clinically significant because bridging fibrosis is more likely to lead to cirrhosis.

All of the scores generated by any of the scoring systems are, by definition, non-parametric and therefore the appropriate statistical tests need to be applied when analysing them. A perusal of the literature will reveal that this has not always been the case!

The question of inter- and intraobserver variation has been examined. The overall conclusion is that for experienced liver pathologists there is reasonably good inter- and intraobserver agreement. Furthermore, the level of agreement is better for fibrosis scores than for inflammation scores. This is encouraging because most people consider the former to be more significant.

Table 2.4
The Ishak (modified HAI) scoring system.

A.   Necroinflammatory score (grade)
Features to be scored
1.   Interface hepatitis (maximum possible score, 4)
2.   Confluent necrosis (maximum possible score, 6)
3.   Lobular inflammation (maximum possible score, 4)
4.   Portal inflammation (maximum possible score, 4)

1 + 2 +3 + 4 = necroinflammatory score (maximum possible score, 18)

B.   Fibrosis (stage)
Normal liver architecture (score, 0) to cirrhosis (maximum possible score, 6)

A liver biopsy takes a sample of an extremely small fraction of the liver's mass. There is also, therefore, a question of sampling error. This has not been as carefully examined as interobserver variation but it does appear that it is a significant problem, especially in hepatitis C, which tends to show more focal changes than hepatitis B. To minimize the effect of sampling error it is important that a liver biopsy should be of adequate size. Although there are no hard data to support this assertion, it is generally accepted that a liver biopsy must have at least three portal tracts before it can be considered large enough. This correlates with a length of approximately 1.5 cm.

It should be remembered that these scoring systems were designed for use in clinical trials, in which the use of a sufficiently large number of biopsies minimizes the impact of these two sources of error. Care must be taken when comparing the scores of just two different biopsies from the same patient, in which the significance of small differences should not be overestimated. Computerized image analysis has been suggested as being an objective means of assessing fibrosis. It should, however, be considered at best complementary to liver biopsy and has no role in routine clinical practice.

To score or not to score

Just because liver biopsies can be scored does not mean that it is always necessary to do so. In the setting of clinical trials where change in histology is one of the end-points it is clearly important to quantify the histological appearance, and the scoring systems were originally designed for this purpose. In routine clinical practice liver biopsy scores may be helpful in those centres that use the scores to determine clinical management but many centres prefer to assess liver biopsies from patients with chronic hepatitis C simply as 'mild', 'moderate' or 'severe' and there is no evidence that this approach is less valuable than formal scoring. Personal preference is probably the most important determinant of whether or not scoring should be used. There is certainly no point in the histopathologist scoring biopsies if the clinician is not going to act on this information.

The role of liver biopsy in the management of chronic hepatitis C

The major role of the liver biopsy in the management of chronic hepatitis C is twofold (Tables 2.5 and 2.6):

- to determine the severity of the liver disease which may be used as one of a number of factors to be considered when determining whether to initiate treatment and to act as a baseline for assessing subsequent disease progression; and
- to determine whether any other disease process is present and to exclude significant iron overload, which may be exacerbated by ribavirin therapy.

The role of liver biopsy management is discussed in more detail in Chapter 3.

Table 2.5
Indications for liver biopsy in chronic hepatitis.

To assess grade and stage
To assess response to treatment
To exclude co-existing causes of liver disease (e.g. haemochromatosis, hepatitis delta virus infection)
To assess dysplasia and malignancy

Table 2.6
A typical liver biopsy report from a patient with hepatitis C virus infection.

Macro
A core of brown tissue 3.1 cm
Micro
Liver with expansion of portal tracts with focal bridging fibrosis. There is moderate portal tract inflammation with poorly formed lymphoid aggregates. Hepatitic bile duct damage is seen, but there is no bile duct loss. There is mild interface hepatitis and moderate lobular inflammation. The latter is associated with moderate large droplet fatty change, but there is no fatty liver hepatitis. Special stains for iron, alpha-1 antitrypsin bodies and copper-associated protein are negative. There is no dysplasia.
Conclusion
A moderate chronic hepatitis with features consistent with hepatitis C virus.
Modified HAI score
Grade – 1+0+2+2=5/18
Stage – 3/6

Further reading

Bartenschlager R, Lohmann V. Replication of hepatitis C virus. *J Gen Virol* 2000; **81**: 1631–48.

Brunt EM. Grading and staging the histopathological lesions of chronic hepatitis: the Knodell histology activity index and beyond. *Hepatology* 2000; **31**: 241–6.

Lefkowitch JH, Schiff ER, Davis GL et al. Pathological diagnosis of chronic hepatitis C: a multicenter comparative study with chronic hepatitis B. The Hepatitis Interventional Therapy Group. *Gastroenterology* 1993; **104**: 595–603.

Monto A. Hepatitis C and steatosis. *Semin Gastrointest Dis* 2002; **13**: 40–6.

Poynard T, Bedossa P, Opolon P. Natural history of liver fibrosis progression in patients with chronic hepatitis C. *Lancet* 1997; **349**: 825–32.

Saadeh S, Cammell G, Carey WD, Younossi Z, Barnes D, Easley K. The role of liver biopsy in chronic hepatitis C. *Hepatology* 2001; **33**: 196–200.

Simmonds P, Holmes EC, Cha TA, et al. Classification of hepatitis C virus into six major genotypes and a series of subtypes by phylogenetic analysis of the NS-5 region. *J Gen Virol* 1993; **74**: 2391–9.

Diagnosis and management of chronic hepatitis C virus infection

3

Patients with chronic hepatitis C virus infection are referred for therapy from a wide variety of healthcare professionals. For all patients who are infected with hepatitis C virus, it is important to confirm the diagnosis and assess the impact of the disease on the patient before planning the therapy.

Diagnosis

Patients who are suspected of having chronic hepatitis C virus infection are normally tested for exposure to hepatitis C virus with an assay that detects antibodies against the virus. A number of different assays are commercially available; some (such as the enzyme immunoassay (EIA)) detect whether antibodies are present or absent while others (such as the recombinant immunoblot assays (RIBA)) identify the antibody target proteins in more detail. RIBA assays usually provide information on the binding of antibodies to four or five antigens from the hepatitis C virus. If two or more are positive, the test indicates exposure to hepatitis C. A single positive is regarded as indeterminate.

Both types of assay, when positive, confirm that the patient has been exposed to the hepatitis C virus. With most viruses, the presence of circulating antibodies indicates past, resolved infection with that virus rather than ongoing infection. This is not the case with the hepatitis C virus – antibodies against the hepatitis C virus are found in patients who are actively infected.

Liver function tests should be done in all patients suspected of having hepatitis C but normal liver function tests do not exclude infection since many infected patients have transiently or persistently normal liver function tests. Equally, the presence of antibodies against hepatitis C virus and abnormal liver function tests do not confirm the diagnosis of chronic hepatitis C virus infection, since another cause for the liver abnormalities may be present. Hence, all patients who have detectable antibodies against the hepatitis C virus should have a sample of serum analysed for the presence of virus by a sensitive assay (usually a polymerase chain reaction (PCR) assay) that is capable of detecting as little as 50 IU/ml (50 IU of virus is approximately equivalent to 100 copies).

A small proportion of patients have detectable antibodies but are persistently 'PCR-negative' – they have undetectable viraemia. In our practice this is unusual and most patients are viraemic at the time of referral. Such patients have presumably been exposed to hepatitis C virus but have eliminated the virus spontaneously. Once this diagnosis has been confirmed no further follow-up is required, but it is important to test the hepatitis C PCR on at least two separate occasions since low level, fluctuating viraemia may confound the diagnosis.

Occasionally, there are patients who do not have detectable antibodies against hepatitis C virus but who are viraemic (i.e. they have detectable hepatitis C virus RNA). This may be seen in patients who are heavily immunosuppressed or who have contracted the infection within the previous few weeks (the antibody response typically takes a few months to develop and hence early infection may be characterized by viraemia in the absence of antibodies). In these patients, a high index of suspicion is required to identify the infection correctly.

Following confirmation of the diagnosis it is important to counsel the patient about infectivity and the effects of the infection on partners and other family members. The issues about transmission of hepatitis C virus are described in detail in Chapter 1, and the natural history of the infection is discussed in Chapter 2. Table 3.1 summarizes the important issues that should be discussed with all infected patients at the time of the diagnosis.

Once the diagnosis of chronic hepatitis C virus infection has been established, a liver biopsy should be considered to grade and stage the disease (see page 30). A liver biopsy was previously considered mandatory prior to commencing antiviral therapy but recent advances in the efficacy of treatment for chronic hepatitis C infection have led many to question the need for a biopsy prior to treatment. Many patients now choose to undergo treatment without undergoing a liver biopsy and this is a reasonable strategy for those who are determined to eliminate the virus as soon as possible. However a liver biopsy provides valuable information about the extent and severity of the disease which cannot be established in any other way, and knowledge of the disease severity plays a central role in deciding the timing of antiviral therapy. The advantages and disadvantages of undergoing a liver biopsy should always be discussed with the patient and, in our experience, the majority prefer to undergo the investigation to allow them to assess the extent of their disease.

Table 3.1
Issues to discuss when counselling a patient with newly diagnosed chronic hepatitis C virus infection.

Issue	Comment
Natural history	Typically slow – only 30% of patients develop cirrhosis after 30 years but difficult to predict progression on an individual basis
Organ/blood donation	Infected patients must not donate
Transmission	
Sex	Risk of sexual transmission is low, less than 3%
Close contact	Transmission risk is nil
Household contact	Very low risk but do not share blood stained items (e.g. toothbrush, razor, etc)
Mother–baby	Transmission risk is less than 5%
Breastfeeding	Transmission risk is nil
Sharing needles and injecting paraphernalia	High risk of transmission – must be avoided
Alcohol	Excess alcohol increases the rate of liver damage and even moderate/light drinking may be harmful
Therapy	Combination therapy cures over 50–60% of infected patients

During the first consultation it is helpful to identify confounding diseases that may complicate therapy and the investigations that should be performed before therapy is started are listed later, in Table 3.7.

Therapy

Modern treatment for chronic hepatitis C infection involves therapy with a long acting ('pegylated') interferon and ribavirin. All clinicians are agreed on the drugs that should be used to treat hepatitis C infection but there is no clear consensus on whether all patients should be treated. Here we will outline the characteristics of the two pegylated interferons before describing their clinical efficacy and discussing the selection of patients for therapy.

The pegylated interferons

The type I interferons are a family of natural cytokines that are produced as part of the innate immune response against viral infections (see page 2). The interferon proteins have been isolated and the genes that encode them have been cloned, so that a variety of type I interferons are now commercially available including:

- recombinant naturally occurring interferons (interferon alfa-2a (Roferon-A) and interferon alfa-2b (Intron));
- recombinant modified interferon (consensus interferon (Infergen)); and
- natural interferons (e.g. Alferon, Sumiferon), which are derived from viral

infection of leucocytes or lymphocytes and which contain several different interferon alpha subtypes.

The natural, unmodified interferons are administered by subcutaneous injection and they have a relatively short half-life of no more than a few hours. To generate reasonable serum concentrations of interferon the conventional interferons need to be administered at least three times a week and this frequent administration is uncomfortable and inconvenient for the patient. Even with thrice weekly injections of conventional interferon there is still marked fluctuation of the serum concentration of interferon and previous attempts to administer the drug more often to reduce these wide variations were only partially successful.

To resolve the problems associated with the short half-life of conventional interferons the interferon protein has been attached to a second molecule, polyethylene glycol, to produce much larger, more stable compounds. Polyethylene glycol (PEG) is an inert chemical that consists of polymerized ethylene glycol chains of varying lengths. When proteins are conjugated to PEG they retain their activity but their serum half-life is increased. Studies in the 1970s with the enzyme adenosine deaminase showed that pegylated enzymes retained activity and could be safely administered to humans. This technology has since been adapted and applied to the type I interferons. At present two pegylated interferons have been developed and both are widely available for the management of patients with chronic hepatitis C.

12KD pegylated interferon alfa-2b (PEG-IFNα2b (12KD))

The first pegylated interferon to be licensed consisted of interferon alfa-2b linked to a 12 kD PEG chain by a cleavable bond that breaks apart when the molecule is added to water. This pegylated interferon is therefore unstable in solution and is supplied as a powder for reconstitution immediately prior to use. Once reconstituted the PEG-IFNα2b (12KD) is administered by subcutaneous injection and, due to its pharmacokinetic characteristics, is given at a dose that is dependent upon the patient's body weight – patients should be weighed and a dose of interferon equal to 1.5 µg/kg administered. Since the PEG-IFNα2b (12KD) is labile in solution it is important that patients administer the entire dose immediately – unused PEG-IFNα2b (12KD) must be discarded because if it is retained the PEG moiety dissociates from the interferon protein and the advantages of pegylation are lost. Following subcutaneous administration the PEG-IFNα2b (12KD) liberates free interferon alfa 2b that is cleared by the kidneys; thus the dose of this pegylated interferon should be adjusted in patients with renal impairment (i.e. patients in whom the glomerular filtration rate is less than 50 ml/min).

40KD pegylated interferon alfa-2a (PEG-IFNα2a (40KD))

The PEG-IFNα2a (40KD) differs significantly from the PEG-IFNα2b (12KD). The PEG moiety that is bound to the interferon is much larger (40 KD rather than 12 KD) and is a branched, rather than a single chain. This leads to much slower absorption, metabolism and excretion of the 40 KD product and the drug therefore has a much longer half-life. In addition, the drug is excreted by both the liver and kidneys and therefore only minor dose adjustments are needed in patients with impaired renal function. Since the bond linking the PEG to the interferon is a stable amide bond that binds to histidine residues this pegylated interferon is stable in solution and therefore does not need to be reconstituted before use. Pharmacological studies have shown that this product does not need to be dosed according to bodyweight and therefore a single, fixed dose (180 µg per week) is suitable for all patients.

The differences between the various interferons are listed in Table 3.2.

Treatment efficacy

Defining 'cure' – lessons from past errors

The early clinical trials for chronic hepatitis C virus infection used interferon alfa monotherapy and led to enthusiastic reports of 'cure' rates approaching 50%. Unfortunately these early trials defined a cure as 'normal liver function tests at the end of therapy', and it soon became clear that many patients with normal liver function tests at the end of therapy went on to relapse during follow-up. Later studies analysed the response to treatment by measuring viral RNA at the end of therapy, and these studies showed that some patients with normal liver function tests remain viraemic, a situation that leads to further distortion of the sustained response rates. Hence early clinical trials used inappropriate end-points and grossly overestimated the proportion of patients who were cured.

Table 3.2
Characteristics of the currently available interferons.

	Conventional interferons	PEG-IFNα2b (12KD)	PEG-IFNα2a (40KD)
Preparation	Ready to inject liquid	Dry powder – requires reconstitution with water before administration	Ready to inject liquid
Administration	Three times a week	Once per week	Once per week
Half-life	Several hours	40 ± 13.3 hours	80 ± 32 hours
Excretion	Predominantly renal	Predominantly renal	Renal and hepatic

The lessons from these early treatment trials have led to the adoption of strict criteria for treatment response and a 'sustained virological response' (SVR) is now defined as the absence of detectable virus 24 weeks after the cessation of therapy. A sensitive PCR test that detects as little as 50 IU/ml of hepatitis C virus RNA must be used. If this strict definition is followed, then patients who show a sustained response to therapy have a greater than 95% chance of remaining non-viraemic with normal liver biochemistry and improved hepatic histology 10 years after the end of therapy. To all intents and purposes these patients are cured, although purists may argue that cure can only be determined when patients have died of a cause that is unrelated to hepatitis C. Occasional relapses many years after therapy do occur (although they are very rare, probably occurring in less than 1% of patients) and may represent reinfection rather than true relapse, and therefore annual follow-up of all treatment responders may be prudent.

For patients who have been cured there is often debate as to whether immunosuppression will lead to viral recurrence (as does occur with hepatitis B virus infection). There are no data to suggest that immuno-suppression may lead to relapse but it would seem wise to continue to monitor these patients until more is known about the long-term outcome.

Efficacy of the pegylated interferons

When used in isolation for 48 weeks (pegylated interferon monotherapy) both of the currently available pegylated interferons are significantly more effective than conventional interferon and the pivotal clinical trials are summarized in Table 3.3.

All interferons used to date have been associated with a wide range of side effects including initial flu-like symptoms (fever, arthralgia, malaise) and later chronic fatigue, weight loss and depression. These side effects are also present with the pegylated interferons but it is clear that the side effects with pegylated interferons are no worse than those seen with conventional interferon and, indeed, some of the adverse effects do seem to be reduced with the long acting interferons. Thus the improvements in response rates that are seen with the pegylated interferons are not associated with an increase in side effects. Clearly pegylated interferons are significantly more effective than conventional interferon, and for patients who are intolerant of ribavirin (see subsequent section) they represent a valuable treatment option.

Ribavirin

Ribavirin is a modified nucleoside analogue that has antiviral activity against a wide range of different viruses. In addition to its antiviral effects, ribavirin can activate Th1 cells and thereby facilitate immunological clearance of an infecting virus (see page 5).

When used as monotherapy for patients with chronic hepatitis C virus infection, ribavirin is disappointing and has no demonstrable antiviral effects, although it may improve the liver function tests by an unidentified mechanism. When ribavirin is combined with interferon in the therapy of

Table 3.3
Efficacy of pegylated interferon monotherapy – sustained virological response rates in the pivotal trials involving pegylated interferon monotherapy

	Conventional interferon	PEG-IFNα2a (40KD)	PEG-IFNα2b (12KD)
All patients	19%	39%	
(Zeuzem et al)[a]	(IFN given at a dose of 6 MIU for 12 weeks followed by 3 MIU for 9 months)		
All patients	12%		25%
(Lindsay et al)[b]	(IFN given at a dose of 3MIU for 12 months)		(Optimal dose was 1 μg per kg)
Patients with cirrhosis	8%	30%	
(Heathcote et al)[c]			

[a] Zeuzem et al. *N Engl J Med* 2000; **343**: 1666–72.
[b] Lindsay et al. *Hepatology* 2001; **34**: 395–403.
[c] Heathcote et al. *N Engl J Med* 2000; **343**: 1673–80.

chronic hepatitis C, the two drugs are synergistic and the combination is markedly more effective than either drug given alone. The mechanism of action of ribavirin in this setting is unclear and it is not known whether the synergistic effects seen with interferon and ribavirin are due to the antiviral activity of ribavirin or to its immunomodulatory properties.

The optimal dose of ribavirin that needs to be combined with interferon has not been exhaustively studied. For patients receiving conventional interferon the doses used are modified by the patient's body weight – for most patients a dose of 1000 mg/day is sufficient but for patients weighing at least 75 kg the dose should be increased to 1200 mg. The dose of ribavirin that should be combined with the pegylated interferons is determined by the genotype and type of pegylated interferon (see later).

Although ribavirin increases the efficacy of interferon therapy it also increases the side effects. Ribavirin induces mild haemolysis that leads to a reduction in the haemoglobin concentration of 2–3 g/dl. This mild anaemia tends to exacerbate the interferon-related malaise, and many patients receiving combination therapy become profoundly fatigued. Recent reports suggest that therapy with erythropoietin may improve the haemoglobin levels in patients receiving ribavirin, but whether this increases compliance, improves outcome and is cost effective has not yet been determined. Ribavirin may induce nausea, a chronic cough and small oral ulcers, and it occasionally causes troublesome dry, scaly skin lesions. Although most patients tolerate these side effects, for some the therapy is intolerable and ribavirin has to be discontinued.

Combination therapy – pegylated interferon and ribavirin

For patients with chronic hepatitis C virus infection, the combination of conventional interferon with ribavirin leads to a significant improvement in the sustained response rate – from 15% to over 40%. The same beneficial effects of ribavirin are seen when it is combined with a pegylated interferon and overall response rates in patients treated with a pegylated interferon and ribavirin are greater than 50%. Data from the two pivotal clinical trials where the two pegylated interferons were compared with conventional interferon and ribavirin are summarized in Tables 3.4 and 3.5.

Table 3.4
Efficacy of PEG-IFNα2b (12KD) and ribavirin.[a]

	Conventional interferon + ribavirin	PEG-IFNα2b (12KD) (low dose) + ribavirin (standard dose)	PEG-IFNα2b (12KD) (high dose) + ribavirin (low dose)
All patients	47%	47%	54%
Genotype 1 all patients	33%	34%	42%
Genotype 1 high viraemia (>800 000 IU/ml)	29%	Not available	30%*
Genotype 2/3	79%	80%	82%

[a]The table lists the proportion of patients who had undetectable hepatitis C viraemia (i.e. were HCV PCR negative) 24 weeks after cessation of therapy.

Note that in this trial two PEG-IFNα2b (12KD) treatment regimens were assessed – one involved a high dose of pegylated interferon (1.5 μg/kg) for 4 weeks followed by a lower dose (0.5 μg/kg) and this was combined with standard dose ribavirin (1000 or 1200 mg depending upon body weight). The second regimen involved a higher dose of pegylated interferon (1.5 μg/kg) plus a lower, fixed dose of ribavirin (800 mg for all patients).

*USA label for PEG-IFNα2b (12KD).
Manns et al. *Lancet* 2001; **358**: 958–65

Table 3.5

Efficacy of the PEG-IFNα2a (40KD) and ribavirin[a]

	Conventional interferon + ribavirin	PEG-IFNα2a (40KD) alone	PEG-IFNα2a (40KD) + ribavirin (standard dose)
All patients	44%	29%	56%
Genotype 1 all patients	36%	21%	46%
Genotype 1 high viraemia (>800 000 IU/ml)	33%	13%	41%
Genotype 2/3	61%	45%	76%

[a]The table lists the proportion of patients who had undetectable HCV viraemia (i.e. were HCV PCR negative) 24 weeks after cessation of therapy).

Fried et al. *N Engl J Med* 2002; **347**: 975–82.

Optimizing the response to therapy with pegylated interferon and ribavirin

The pivotal clinical trials show that the combination of pegylated interferon and ribavirin is more effective than conventional interferon. However, these trials studied a limited number of different ribavirin doses and all patients were treated for 48 weeks. Hence firm conclusions about the optimal dose of ribavirin and the optimal duration of therapy can not be made from these studies. For the PEG-IFNα2a (40KD) a follow-up clinical study assessed the efficacy of different doses of ribavirin and different durations of therapy. This study showed that for this pegylated interferon patients with hepatitis C virus of genotypes 2 and 3 need only 24 weeks of therapy with ribavirin at a dose of 800 mg per day and this regimen leads to sustained virological response rates that are identical to those seen with longer treatment durations and higher doses. For patients with genotype 1 hepatitis C shortening the treatment duration and/or reducing the dose of ribavirin led to a decrease in efficacy. Hence for this pegylated interferon the recommendation is that patients with genotype 1 receive 48 weeks therapy with standard dose ribavirin and that patients with genotypes 2 and 3 receive 24 weeks therapy with low dose ribavirin (800 mg) (see Table 3.6).

Table 3.6
Efficacy of the PEG-IFNα2a (40KD) and ribavirin tested at different doses and different treatment durations. The table lists the proportion of patients who had undetectable HCV viraemia (i.e. were HCV PCR negative) 24 weeks after cessation of therapy.

	PEG-IFNα2a (40KD) + 800 mg ribavirin for 24 weeks	PEG-IFNα2a (40KD) + 1000/1200 mg ribavirin for 24 weeks	PEG-IFNα2a (40KD) + 800 mg ribavirin for 48 weeks	PEG-IFNα2a (40KD) + 1000/1200 mg ribavirin for 48 weeks
All patients				63%
Genotype 1	29%	42%	41%	52%
Genotype 1 with high level viraemia	16%	26%	36%	47%
Genotype 1 with low level viraemia	41%	52%	55%	65%
Genotype 2 and 3	84%	81%	79%	80%

Data from Hadziyannis et al. *Ann Intern Med* 2004; **140**: 346–55.

The highlighted boxes indicate the recommended doses

For the PEG-IFNα2b (12KD) a recent clinical trial examined the effects of 24 weeks of therapy in patients with hepatitis C virus of genotypes 2 and 3. This single arm study involved a comparison with historical controls and showed that, like the PEG-IFNα2a (40KD), this pegylated interferon should be used for 24 weeks in patients infected with these, treatment sensitive, viral genotypes. However, this trial also showed that for the PEG-IFNα2b (12KD) patients with genotype 2 and 3 require high doses of ribavirin that are adjusted for body weight – patients weighing less than 65 kg should receive 800 mg, patients weighing 65–85 kg should receive 1000 mg, patients weighing 85–105 kg should receive 1200 mg and heavier patients should receive 1400 mg, although these dosing regimens are not yet included in the licensed dosing schedules. Furthermore the results with the PEG-IFNα2b (12KD) and ribavirin suggest that patients with genotype 3 and high level viraemia have a reduced response when compared to patients with genotype 3 and low level viraemia, perhaps suggesting that such patients may benefit from longer courses of therapy with the PEG-IFNα2b (12KD) and ribavirin, although this approach has not yet been formally tested.

Thus for patients infected with hepatitis C virus of genotype 2 or 3 there are important differences in the doses of ribavirin that need to be administered with the different pegylated interferons – patients receiving the PEG-IFNα2a (40KD), require 800 mg of ribavirin per day and patients receiving the PEG-IFNα2b (12KD) require a dose of ribavirin that is modified according to body weight (800–1400 mg/day).

For patients with hepatitis C virus of genotype 1 who are receiving the PEG-IFNα2b (12KD) the most appropriate dose of ribavirin and the optimal duration of therapy have not yet been assessed in prospective clinical trials. The pivotal trials with the optimal dose of PEG-IFNα2b (12KD) (1.5 μg/kg) used a fixed dose of ribavirin (800 mg) and retrospective analysis of the results indicated that light weight patients had better response rates than heavier patients. One explanation for this is that light weight patients may have had higher serum concentrations of ribavirin and it is plausible that this contributed to their improved response rates. This led to the hypothesis that increasing the dose of ribavirin in heavier patients would improve response rates and it is therefore recommended that patients receiving the PEG-IFNα2b (12KD) are treated with a dose of ribavirin depending upon body weight – patients weighing less than 65 kg should receive 800 mg, patients weighing 65–85 kg should receive 1000 mg, patients weighing 85–105 kg should receive 1200 mg and heavier patients should receive 1400 mg. These doses have not yet been assessed in clinical trials for patients with genotype 1 infection and are not currently included in the drug license.

Large scale controlled clinical trials examining the response rates and optimal duration of therapy with hepatitis C virus genotypes other than 1, 2 and 3 have not been completed. For patients with genotype 4 infection small scale clinical trials with PEG-IFNα2a (40KD) and ribavirin suggest that 48 weeks of therapy with standard doses of ribavirin are required but that response rates of >70% may be expected.

Early cessation of therapy – stopping ineffective treatment

The effectiveness of combination therapy with the pegylated interferons can be assessed after only 12 weeks of therapy. If the patient has not lost virus after 12 weeks of therapy (i.e. hepatitis C virus testing shows that the virus is still present) or if the level of circulating viraemia (assessed by quantitative testing) has not fallen by at least 100-fold (a 2 log drop) then the patient has a very low probability (less than 3%) of responding to therapy. Hence unsuccessful therapy with the pegylated interferons and ribavirin can be discontinued after 3 months, sparing patients the side effects of prolonged therapy. However, the proportion of patients with genotypes 2 and 3 who do not respond after 12 weeks is extremely small and therefore most clinicians do not test patients with these genotypes as the number of patients who are identified is extremely small (<5%).

Predicting the response to therapy

The major determinant of the response to therapy for patients with chronic hepatitis C is the viral genotype and this variable dominates all of the response rates. However, a number of other factors have been identified that influence the treatment outcome. Patients with high level viraemia respond less well to therapy than those with low viral loads, and concurrent alcohol intake significantly reduces the response to therapy. Additional factors that influence the response to therapy are the degree of fibrosis (patients with cirrhosis have a significant reduction in their response to treatment) and the serum alanine aminotransferase (ALT) at the start of therapy – patients with higher levels of ALT respond more effectively than those with lower levels, perhaps indicating that the level of inflammatory activity reflects immune responses to the virus. A patient's age has a marked effect on the response – older patients respond less well than do younger patients and obesity reduces the response rates. Hence the ideal patient is young, thin with low level viraemia, minimal fibrosis and genotype non-1.

Management during pegylated interferon and ribavirin therapy

Pretreatment assessment (Table 3.7)

It is essential that all fertile women planning to start ribavirin should be screened for pregnancy before therapy and all should be taking adequate contraceptive precautions. Past experience convinces us that 'careful abstinence' in single women is not effective contraception and we insist that all women of childbearing age take regular contraceptives or carry condoms at all times. Since ribavirin has a long half-life, effective contraception should be continued for at least 6 months after therapy. It is important that all men planning to commence therapy take effective contraceptive precautions for the duration of therapy and for a further 6 months after therapy.

All patients should be carefully assessed before starting combination therapy. The full blood count should be reviewed and patients who are anaemic (haemoglobin <11 g/dl), thrombocytopenic (platelet count $<70 \times 10^9$ cells/l) or neutropenic (neutrophil count $<1 \times 10^9$ cells/l) should not normally be commenced on combination therapy. In patients over the age of 40, a chest radiograph and electrocardiogram (ECG) are prudent to exclude significant pulmonary and cardiac disease that may be exacerbated by ribavirin-associated anaemia. The hepatological investigations should always be reviewed before therapy to confirm the diagnosis, and thyroid function should be evaluated.

One of the most feared complications of interferon therapy is suicidal depression, probably related to an interferon-induced reduction in serotonin levels in the central nervous system.

Characteristically the patient becomes profoundly depressed and loses insight such that the cause of the depression (interferon therapy) is not apparent. All patients receiving interferon should be assessed before therapy to determine the likelihood of severe depression. A past history of

Table 3.7
Investigations that should be done prior to starting therapy for patients with chronic hepatitis C infection.

Investigation	Comment
Hepatitis C RNA PCR	Confirms the diagnosis. The level of viraemia (quantitative PCR) is helpful, particularly in patients with genotype 1
Hepatitis B serology	If co-infection with hepatitis B is confirmed consider alternative treatment approaches
HIV	Should be considered in all patients and, if the patient is regarded as high risk testing for HIV co-infection should be performed after appropriate consent
Liver function tests	Important baseline investigation
Renal function	Impaired renal function may require dose of ribavirin to be adjusted
Full blood count	
Haemoglobin	Likely to fall by 2–3 gm during therapy
White cell count	Will decrease during therapy
Platelet count	Will decrease during therapy
Thyroid function tests	May deteriorate during therapy
Serum ferritin	If markedly raised (>3 times the upper limit normal) indicates iron overload which may impair the response to therapy
Autoantibodies	If present at a titre >1:80 reconsider the diagnosis
Pregnancy test	Ribavirin is contraindicated in pregnant women
ECG	For patients at risk of significant heart disease
Chest radiograph	For patients at risk of significant heart and lung disease

psychiatric disease requiring hospitalization may indicate an increased risk, and such patients should not normally receive interferon therapy. Patients who have received outpatient antidepressant therapy in the past may be treated with interferon but vigilance is required, and it may be wise to consider starting such patients on prophylactic antidepressant medication before starting therapy.

Management during therapy

Combination therapy with conventional interferon and ribavirin can be very unpleasant and is associated with a very significant reduction in an individual's quality of life that lasts throughout the duration of therapy. Although the pegylated interferons do cause some interferon-related side effects their frequency and severity is reduced when compared to conventional

Faced with a slowly progressive disease and unpleasant, poorly effective therapy many patients and clinicians decided to defer therapy in individuals with mild hepatitis C hoping that more effective and more palatable treatments would become available before they had developed significant liver disease. This led to the development of biopsy-based management algorithms in which all patients with chronic hepatitis C were advised to have a liver biopsy and therapy was only recommended for those with moderate/severe disease – usually defined as a fibrosis score of greater than 2 and a necroinflammatory score of 4 or more on the Knodell classification. This approach proved popular with patients and was widely adopted.

The development of the pegylated inteferons, which are more effective and better tolerated than the conventional interferons, has led to a re-evaluation of the biopsy-based management approach. For patients with genotype 2 or 3 hepatitis C infection the very good response to pegylated interferon and ribavirin (>75% of patients respond to therapy) and the short duration of treatment and low dose ribavirin with the PEG-IFNα2a (40KD) has led us to consider treating patients with mild infection and therefore a liver biopsy is no longer necessary for patients who are infected with these genotypes. However, knowledge of the severity of the liver disease plays an important role in patient motivation – individuals with moderate disease are more inclined to tolerate the side effects of therapy than those who have minimal fibrosis and therefore we presently advise patients with genotype 2 or 3 hepatitis C infection to

undergo a liver biopsy. However, in patients who do not wish to have a biopsy, or have a contraindication to the procedure, we do commence treatment without insisting that the biopsy be performed.

For patients with hepatitis C of genotype 1 infection the longer duration of therapy (48 weeks) and the reduced response rates indicate that patients with mild disease may be best advised to defer therapy until more effective treatments are available. Hence a liver biopsy remains a key investigation in these patients. However, some patients with genotype 1 chronic infection and minimal disease still wish to undergo treatment and, as always, the patient should be allowed to make the final decision as to whether or not to undergo therapy. If therapy is deferred then it is important to monitor the patient and to repeat the liver biospy in 3–5 years time to ensure that the disease has not progressed. If the repeat liver biopsy shows disease progression then therapy should be instituted.

Complex cases: controversial management issues

Previous treatment failure

The widespread use of conventional interferon and ribavirin has led to an increasing group of patients who present after having failed an initial course of therapy. The optimal management of this group of patients is not yet clear but studies to date indicate that for patients who have failed to respond to conventional interferon monotherapy there is a reasonable chance of a sustained virological response (around 30%) when these patients are re-treated with a pegylated interferon and ribavirin. For patients who have had a partial response to conventional interferon and ribavirin (i.e. lost virus for a period of time during a course of therapy) around 40–60% may respond to pegylated interferon and ribavirin. However, the response rates are somewhat lower in patients who have failed to respond to conventional interferon and ribavirin and only 10–20% respond to therapy with a pegylated interferon. At present we offer therapy to those who have failed to respond to conventional interferon and ribavirin and the majority of patients are willing to try again. Studies of novel therapeutic regimens to increase efficacy in previous non responders are awaited with interest.

There is some early evidence to suggest that long-term maintenance interferon therapy may reduce the progression of liver fibrosis and prevent the development of liver cancer and a National Institute of Health supported study involving 90 µg of the PEG-IFNα2a (40KD) given for several years is currently underway to address this important issue.

Active drug users

Many patients with chronic hepatitis C virus infection have a past history of injecting drug use and some are actively using drugs when they are referred for therapy. For patients receiving methadone replacement therapy there is good evidence to show that compliance with antiviral therapy is good and the sustained response rates are similar to those seen in other patient groups. There is widespread agreement that these patients should be

treated. However, anecdotal reports suggest that patients who have recently withdrawn from methadone therapy may relapse when exposed to the rigours of combination therapy, and our policy is to treat patients who are receiving maintenance methadone rather than waiting for the patient to withdraw completely from opiates.

For patients who are actively using non-prescribed 'street' drugs a number of small scale studies have shown that compliance with antiviral therapy is good and re-infection in those who eliminate the virus is very rare. Hence these patients should be considered for antiviral therapy. However, many such patients have other, more pressing, healthcare concerns and the majority of active drug users decline therapy when it is offered to them. It is important to ensure that these individuals receive appropriate lifestyle advice and support; for those who do decide to try therapy, treatment with a pegylated interferon and ribavirin is often successful and this has the added advantage of reducing the number of infected individuals who may transmit the virus to others.

Associated liver autoantibodies

Chronic hepatitis C virus infection is occasionally associated with liver autoantibodies. In such patients the question arises as to whether the autoantibodies are coincidental or whether they are contributing to the liver damage. In some patients the histology provides a clue, but in many the dominant disease is not clear. Unusually large numbers of plasma cells and particularly active interface hepatitis suggest that autoimmune liver disease is the dominant problem (Figure 3.1), but the diagnosis is rarely clear-cut.

In these patients, therapy with prednisolone (for a presumed autoimmune disease) improves the liver function regardless of the underlying disease. However, if the primary cause of the liver damage is infection with hepatitis C virus, the improvement in liver function may be associated with progression of the hepatic fibrosis. If these patients are treated with interferon and the main cause of the liver damage is immmuological, then the interferon induces a rapid deterioration in liver function – interferon withdrawal followed by immunosuppression is then the appropriate management option.

Hence, we recommend that these patients are commenced on interferon therapy to determine whether their primary hepatic disease is viral or immunological and, during this therapeutic trial, liver function should be monitored closely. If the liver function

tests show improvement, the liver disease is probably viral in origin, and antiviral therapy should be continued; if the levels of serum transaminases rise, autoimmune disease is likely, and interferon should be withdrawn and therapy with prednisolone considered. These patients should be closely monitored by serial liver biopsies since progression of the fibrosis may occur.

Children

The natural history of chronic hepatitis C virus infection in children has not yet been defined – small-scale studies suggest that the disease is likely to be mild during the first few years after infection but the long-term outlook is not clear and clearly the lifetime risk of liver complications must be considerable. Few clinical trials have been performed in children, and in view of the slow natural history in young people it is probably appropriate to treat children only in the context of controlled clinical trials.

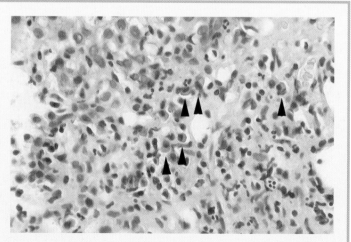

Figure 3.1
Liver biopsy from a patient with hepatitis C virus infection. The inflammatory infiltrate contains conspicuous plasma cells, which is unusual and raises the possibility of an autoimmune hepatitis.

Normal ALT

Many patients with chronic hepatitis C infection have persistently normal liver function tests and over a period of many months serial measurements of serum ALT show that the ALT never increases to more than the upper limit of normal. Such patients may have liver biopsy evidence of significant disease although many have histologically mild disease. In the past these patients were regarded as a special group with disease that did not require therapy and, indeed, some early studies with conventional interferons suggested that such patients might develop deranged liver function tests when treated (i.e. there was evidence for a deterioration in liver function tests after starting therapy). Such patients have traditionally been denied therapy and excluded from clinical trials.

A recent randomized controlled clinical trial with the PEG-IFNα2a (40KD) shows that patients with 'normal ALT' respond very well to therapy with PEG-IFNα2a (40KD) and ribavirin and sustained response rates are similar to those seen in patients with abnormal LFTs. Interestingly, many patients with so-called 'normal ALT' had a reduction in their ALT following viral eradication suggesting that a 'normal ALT' does not necessarily imply that there is no on-going liver damage. Hence, current studies show that the serum ALT is a very poor predictor of liver disease and patients with normal liver function tests should be offered therapy in the same way that patients with abnormal LFTs should be considered as candidates for treatment.

Acute hepatitis C infection

Occasionally patients who have recently contracted hepatitis C are seen – typically such patients present with an episode of jaundice but occasionally asymptomatic individuals are seen, for example following occupational exposure to hepatitis C. Studies to date indicate that if such patients are treated within the first 6 months of infection with conventional interferon monotherapy the response to therapy is excellent with response rates approaching 90%. Although trials with the pegylated interferons in these patients have not been performed it is likely that they will be equally, or even more effective, and in view of their ease of administration these long acting interferons should be used. There is an ongoing debate as to whether to initiate therapy immediately such patients are seen or whether to defer therapy for a few weeks to determine whether or not the patient will eradicate the virus spontaneously. Our current practice is to observe patients for no more than 8 weeks and if the virus becomes undetectable we defer therapy and keep the patient under review. For patients who do not show signs of eliminating the virus spontaneously we advocate therapy with pegylated interferon monotherapy for 6 months, although this advice may change when data from ongoing clinical trials become available.

Further reading

Foster GR. Management of chronic hepatitis C – time for a change? *J Viral Hepat* 2002; **9**: 82–3.

Fried M et al. Peginterferon alfa-2a plus ribavirin for chronic hepatitis C virus infection. *N Engl J Med* 2002; **347**: 975–82.

Lauer GM, Walker BD. Hepatitis C infection. *N Engl J Med* 2001; **345**: 41–52.

McHutchison JG, Gordon SC, Schiff ER, et al. Interferon alfa-2b alone or in combination with ribavirin as initial treatment for chronic hepatitis C. Hepatitis Interventional Therapy Group. *N Engl J Med* 1998; **339**: 1485–92.

Manns MP et al. Peginterferon alfa-2b plus ribavirin compared with interferon alfa-2b plus ribavirin for initial treatment of chronic hepatitis C: a randomised trial. *Lancet* 2001; **358**: 958–65.

Strader DB et al. Diagnosis, management and treatment of hepatitis C. *Hepatology* 2004; **39**: 1147–74.

Questions

1. In the diagnosis of chronic hepatitis C virus infection:
   A. The presence of antibodies against the virus indicates past infection
   B. Normal liver function tests indicate that the virus has been eliminated
   C. A sensitive test that detects 50 IU/ml of hepatitis C virus RNA should be used in all patients
   D. Quantification of the hepatitis C virus RNA titre is not necessary to confirm the diagnosis
   E. Patient counselling increases patient anxiety and should be avoided

2. Ribavirin therapy for patients with chronic hepatitis C virus infection:
   A. Should be given by intramuscular injection
   B. Induces a haemolytic anaemia that may respond to therapy with erythropoietin
   C. Is effective as monotherapy
   D. Should not normally be used at doses of less than 600 mg
   E. Synergizes with interferon by activating Th2 type responses

3. Combination therapy with interferon and ribavirin in patients with chronic hepatitis C:
   A. Is the treatment of choice
   B. May cure over 50% of patients when a pegylated interferon is used
   C. Can be used in pregnant women to reduce the risks of maternal–fetal transmission
   D. May induce permanent thyroid disease
   E. Requires regular assessment of white cell count and platelet count

4. Combination therapy for chronic hepatitis C virus infection:
   A. Should be offered to patients with depression as viral clearance may improve fatigue-like symptoms
   B. May require antidepressant therapy during treatment to reduce the drug related side effects
   C. Is ineffective in patients with cirrhosis
   D. Should be offered to patients with mild liver disease because response rates are higher in this group of patients
   E. Should be avoided in patients with severe ischaemic heart disease

Answers

Question 1

A. False – in chronic hepatitis C virus infection antibodies co-exist with the virus and hence the presence of antibodies usually indicates ongoing infection
B. False – liver function tests may be normal even in the presence of significant liver disease
C. True
D. True
E. False

Question 2

A. False – the drug should be used orally
B. True
C. False
D. True – in patients of average weight, doses less than 600 mg are probably ineffective
E. False. the drug synergizes by activating Th1 responses

Question 3

A. True
B. True
C. False – ribavirin is teratogenic and must be avoided in pregnant women
D. True
E. True

Question 4

A. False – interferon may aggravate pre-existing depression and carries a substantial risk of suicide in those with previous psychiatric disorders
B. True
C. False – response rates are reduced in patients with cirrhosis but a significant proportion of patients will respond
D. False
E. True

Hepatitis B – virology, natural history and pathology

4

The hepatitis B virus is an unusual virus – it is one of the smallest human pathogens and yet it causes more chronic infections than any other virus. The hepatitis B viral genome was first sequenced in 1979 but the functions of some of the encoded proteins are still unclear. Like the hepatitis C virus and HIV, the hepatitis B virus mutates at a high rate and, as the disease progresses, new viral species develop that lead to different forms of the disease. Recent therapeutic developments involve nucleoside analogues that target the hepatitis B virus directly. These drugs significantly modify the course of chronic infection and may lead to the production of mutant viral strains with different characteristics.

Hepatitis B – the virus

Hepatitis B virus belongs to the Hepadnaviridae viral family. Other members of this group infect birds (such as Peking ducks and herons) as well as small rodents (such as woodchucks), and the availability of these small animal models of infection has greatly facilitated studies into the pathogenesis of the human form of hepatitis B virus infection. The virus is distantly related to the retroviruses that cause immunodeficiency syndromes, and the polymerase protein that duplicates the hepatitis B genome is sufficiently similar to the HIV polymerase for some drugs to inhibit both enzymes and act against both viruses.

The hepatitis B virus is a very small virus – the whole genome is only 3.2 kb long (i.e. the DNA that makes up the entire virus is smaller than some human genes). To compress all the information needed to produce an infectious agent into this very small genome, hepatitis B virus uses 'overlapping open reading frames' to encode the four proteins that make up the intact virus (Figure 4.1). This overlapping genomic structure allows the hepatitis B

Figure 4.1
Schematic diagram of the hepatitis B virus. The partially double-stranded DNA genome encodes four open reading frames. The surface gene contains three initiation codons that lead to the production of three different proteins (preS1, preS2 and surface protein) with different amino terminals but a common carboxy domain. These three proteins form both the envelope of the virus and the 'empty' virus particles (HBsAg). The core gene has two initiation codons that lead to the production of the core protein itself or a truncated, soluble version (HBeAg).

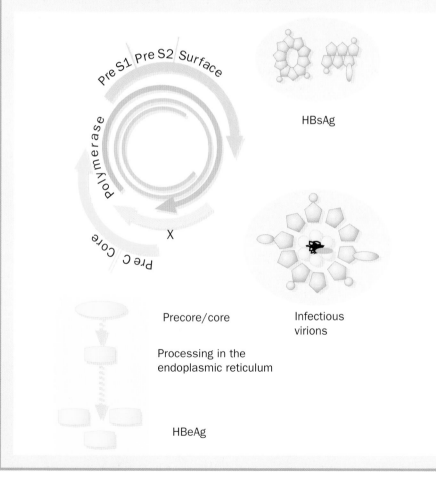

virus to pack a large amount of genetic material into a very small genetic space. However, because many DNA bases code for more than one amino acid, many mutations are non-viable because they lead to the production of defective proteins. This is easily seen by examining the overlap between the envelope protein of hepatitis B virus (the surface protein) and the polymerase protein. These two proteins use the same DNA sequence to encode different proteins but any change to the surface protein leads to a change in the polymerase protein. Hence hepatitis B virus cannot readily mutate its envelope (unlike hepatitis C virus) because many changes in the surface protein have an impact on the polymerase and lead to the production of non-functional viruses. Likewise only a few mutations in the polymerase protein are permitted since many changes lead to the generation of defective viral envelopes.

The replication of hepatitis B virus has been studied in tissue culture models, and the details are now well established (Figure 4.2). The virus enters a cell and releases its partially double-stranded DNA genome. This genome is converted to covalently closed, circular DNA (cccDNA), which acts both as an infectious reservoir and as a template for replication. Some of the cccDNA remains in the nucleus, where it acts as a non-replicating viral repository that is unaffected by antiviral drugs. The remainder of the cccDNA is used to produce an RNA intermediate – the pregenomic RNA. This RNA is then reverse transcribed by the hepatitis B virus polymerase protein (POL) to produce new DNA that is ultimately duplicated and packaged into new viral particles.

During the replication cycle, new viral proteins are produced and combined to produce new virions. Some of the hepatitis B virus proteins are produced in excess and exported out of the cell to form circulating viral proteins that lack any viral nucleic acid. The hepatitis B virus surface protein is produced in vast excess and the released proteins form circulating particles whose function is not clear. These 'empty' viral particles, which contain only the hepatitis B virus surface proteins, are easily detected by standard laboratory assays and they form the basis of the hepatitis B virus surface antigen (HBsAg) diagnostic assay. Hence the assay that is widely used to detect hepatitis B virus infection actually identifies 'empty' viral shells and not the infectious virus.

The hepatitis B virus core protein is normally enclosed within the virus proper. However, the hepatitis B virus core gene can also be translated to produce a larger protein (precore–core), and this protein enters the endoplasmic reticulum, where it is cleaved to produce a smaller protein, HBeAg. This protein is secreted into the circulation, where it may be tolerogenic (see page 7). In clinical practice, HBeAg is a very useful marker of viral replication – its presence indicates that the virus is replicating at a high level and that the patient's serum will contain large numbers of infectious virions. In general, immune responses against HBeAg are associated with responses against other viral proteins and are associated with a reduction in the level of viral replication.

In addition to the two structural proteins (surface and core), the hepatitis B virus genome encodes two non-structural

Figure 4.2
Replication of the hepatitis B virus. (A) After entry into the cell (B) the virus is uncoated and (C) the partially double-stranded DNA is released. (D) The partially double-stranded DNA is transported to the nucleus where it is converted to cccDNA. This cccDNA may remain in the nucleus to form a reservoir of non-replicating DNA, but most of the cccDNA is used as a template for the production of pregenomic RNA. (E) This pregenomic RNA acts as a template for the polymerase protein that converts the RNA into DNA (reverse transcription) before being destroyed by the polymerase-associated RNase. (F, G) The new DNA is converted into the partially double stranded DNA form and then packaged into new virions before release.

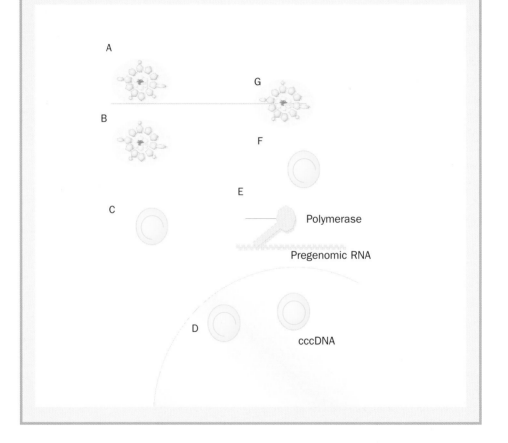

proteins – the X and POL proteins. The functions of the X protein are still unclear but it appears to play a role in regulating viral replication by controlling transcription of the viral genome. The complex POL protein contains the enzymes required for viral replication, including a reverse transcriptase and an RNase, and these combine to replicate the viral genome (see Figure 4.2).

There are seven known HBV genotypes, distinguished by a divergence greater than 8% in the entire genomic sequence, which are designated A to G. These genotypes have relatively distinct geographic distributions: A predominates in North-western Europe, North America, and Africa; B and C are more common in Asia, D is the most common in the Mediterranean countries, E is restricted to West Africa, and F is localized in the New World. These HBV variants have been shown to vary in terms of the host immune recognition, enhanced virulence with increased replication of HBV, resistance to antiviral therapies. For example in one study, genotypes A and C were associated with a higher prevalence of HBeAg compared to genotypes B and D, and genotype D patients were more likely to have decompensated cirrhosis. Nevertheless, genotyping has no current role to play in routine clinical practice.

Natural history of chronic hepatitis B virus infection

The hepatitis B virus replicates almost exclusively in hepatocytes. Cells that are infected with the virus tolerate the infection remarkably well, and infected cells are usually not damaged by the virus. Hence many patients can sustain very large amounts of replicating virus without any significant liver injury.

Natural history of perinatally acquired chronic hepatitis B

The various phases of chronic hepatitis B virus infection are shown in Figure 4.3.

Immunotolerant phase of hepatitis B virus infection

In most countries, chronic hepatitis B virus infection is acquired early in life, either during birth or in the first few years of life. After infection, there is a reduced host response to the virus and the virus replicates at high level. It is not known why the host immune system does not recognize or respond to the presence of the virus but transplacental passage of HBeAg is believed to play a role in inducing a state of immunological tolerance in some patients. During this early 'immunotolerant' phase of hepatitis B virus infection, HBsAg and HBeAg are found in high concentration in the serum, and up to 10^9 copies/ml of hepatitis B virus DNA can be detected. Since there is no immune response against the virus there is no liver inflammation, and the liver function tests are usually normal or near normal.

Immunoactive phase of hepatitis B virus infection

In most patients the immune system eventually recognizes the foreign virus and an immune response develops. This leads to an increase in liver cell damage (and an increase in serum aminotransferase levels). During this second phase – the immunoactive phase – the evolving immune response either controls the infection and the disease remits, or the immune response leads to a prolonged period of hepatic inflammation that often leads to cirrhosis.

Hence, during the immunoactive phase the liver is either killed or cured! If the

Figure 4.3
The natural history of chronic hepatitis B virus infection. Shortly after infection, the virus replicates at high levels, but there is no effective immune response (immunotolerance phase) and there is little hepatic damage. A variable time after infection, an immune response against the virus develops and leads to an increase in the severity of the liver damage, which may progress to cirrhosis at this stage. The immune response usually suppresses the viral replication, and the level of circulating viraemia declines and HBeAg is lost from the serum. This immunosurveillance phase may persist for many years but in some patients the virus mutates and disease develops once again. ALT, alanine aminotransferase.

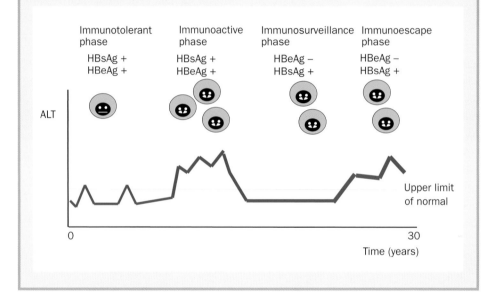

immune response against hepatitis B virus is sufficient to control the virus, there is often a brief increase in the hepatic inflammation during the elimination process, and this is usually associated with the loss of HBeAg and the development of antibodies against HBeAg. This 'seroconversion hepatitis' usually marks the transition from high-level viral replication to low-level viral replication, and the level of viraemia falls markedly (usually to less than 10^5 copies/ml serum). Although HBeAg is eliminated, HBsAg persists.

If the immune response fails to control the infection, there is a prolonged period of fluctuating serum transaminase levels associated with increasing liver damage. The serum virological markers show that both HBsAg and HBeAg persist, and hepatitis B virus DNA may be detected at high levels (10^6–10^9 copies/ml). Since the liver injury is due to the immune response, there is no correlation between the level of viraemia and the severity of the hepatitis.

Immunosurveillance phase of hepatitis B virus infection

If the immunoactive phase of hepatitis B virus infection leads to control of the virus, the patient enters the immunosurveillance phase. During this phase of the infection the patient has:

- low levels of circulating virus;
- undetectable HBeAg; and
- readily detectable HBsAg.

Since the levels of circulating virus are low, the patient is of low infectivity and transmission of the virus to others is extremely rare. The patient may be regarded as having 'hepatitis B surface antigenaemia'. Patients in this phase of hepatitis B virus infection used to be referred to as 'chronic asymptomatic carriers'. However, since most phases of hepatitis B virus infection are asymptomatic and since patients during this phase of the infection are not actually carrying the virus, the term is unhelpful and is best avoided.

The natural history of the immuno-surveillance phase of chronic hepatitis B virus infection is not yet clear. A small proportion of patients go on to eliminate all traces of the virus and HBsAg eventually disappears from the serum along with all other circulating viral proteins. These patients may be regarded as 'cured', although severe immunosuppression (e.g. during chemotherapy) may lead to a relapse.

Immunoescape chronic hepatitis B (HBeAg negative chronic hepatitis B)

Unfortunately, in a significant proportion of patients with hepatitis B surface antigenaemia, the virus becomes active again (immunoescape chronic hepatitis B). In these patients the level of hepatitis B virus DNA in the serum rises (usually above 10^5 copies/ml) and the hepatitis recurs with an increase in the level of the serum transaminases. The HBeAg remains undetectable and the antibodies against HBeAg persist. Careful analysis of the virus during this phase of the infection invariably reveals mutant viruses that lack the ability to produce HBeAg. The most common mutation causing this relapse is a mutation in the precore region that leads to a failure to produce the HBeAg. Hence this form of hepatitis B is often referred to as 'precore mutant hepatitis B'. However, in some viral strains the precore mutant is unstable; in such strains mutations in the core promoter lead to the replication of viruses in the absence of HBeAg, so the term 'precore mutant hepatitis B' may be inaccurate and is probably best avoided.

HBeAg-negative chronic hepatitis B is becoming the dominant form of the disease in many countries, and its management is often problematic (see page 95).

Adult-acquired hepatitis B

Adults who are infected with the hepatitis B virus usually develop an acute, self-limiting illness. The patient becomes jaundiced and unwell, with upper abdominal pain. Joint aches are common. In most patients the illness resolves without sequelae, but in a small minority (2%) the disease leads on to acute liver failure (fulminant hepatitis). Early detection of acute liver failure is essential for successful management (usually

Figure 4.6
*Immunohisto-
chemical stain for
HBsAg, which
confirms that the
ground glass
change is due to
the accumulation
of HBsAg in the
cytoplasm.*

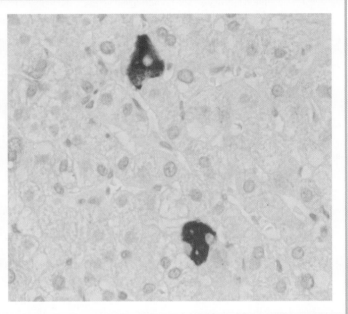

Figure 4.7
*Hepatocytes with
intensely pink
granular cytoplasm
caused by the
accumulation of
large numbers of
mitochondria. This
change can be
seen in many types
of liver damage.*

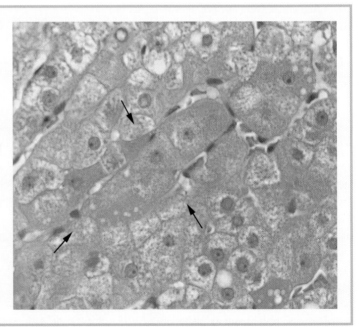

B virus DNA into the genome of the cell and its subsequent transcription. Ground glass cells can be demonstrated by histochemical techniques (Gamori's aldehyde fuschin, orcein or Victoria blue stain) or by immunohistochemical techniques.

There are other, unusual causes of ground glass cells, the most common of which is induction of the smooth endoplasmic reticulum by enzyme-inducing drugs; other causes include Lafora bodies in myoclonic epilepsy and fibrinogen storage disease.

Ground glass cells also need to be distinguished from cells showing oxyntic change. Oxyntic change can be seen both in chronic hepatitis B and hepatitis C (Figure 4.7). This is a form of cellular degeneration in which the cells come to contain large numbers of closely packed mitochondria.

In the very rare cases in which ground glass hepatocytes on liver biopsy are seen but in which the patient is serum HBsAg-negative, immunohistochemical staining is useful. Ground glass cells are especially prominent in patients with immunotolerant hepatitis B with relatively inactive disease. In the immunoactive phase of chronic hepatitis B, the liver damage is due to immunological injury by cytotoxic CD8-positive T lymphocytes that recognize HBeAg or HBcAg on the surface of infected hepatocytes in association with HLA class 1 antigens (see page 5). The histological correlate of this is that lymphocytes are often seen in close relation to damaged hepatocytes. The presence of marked lobular inflammation and cytopathic liver cell damage with hepatocytes that show acidophilic

degeneration in a patient with chronic hepatitis B should always raise the possibility of superimposed hepatitis delta virus infection (see page 100).

Chronic hepatitis B virus infection is frequently associated with large cell dysplasia (change), which is a marker for an increased risk of developing liver cell cancer (see page 140). Given the frequency of hepatitis B virus infection in certain ethnic groups, the presence of another cause of liver disease should always be considered. The exclusion of other causes of liver disease is one reason why many clinicians feel that all patients with chronic viral hepatitis should have at least one liver biopsy.

Immunohistochemical features of chronic hepatitis B virus infection

A wide range of commercially available antibodies to hepatitis B virus are available. While there are cases in which immunohistochemical staining of liver biopsies is valuable, such cases are uncommon and many laboratories frequently carry out staining for hepatitis B virus antigens unnecessarily. This is because immunohistochemical staining rarely provides information not already available from serology. There are a number of circumstances in which immunohistochemical staining can be useful; these are discussed below and summarized in Table 4.2. As discussed above, cytoplasmic HBsAg staining is seen in ground glass hepatocytes. Membranous and submembranous staining can also be seen (see Figure 4.5). Membranous staining correlates with active viral replication. Both HBcAg and HBeAg produce nuclear

Table 4.2
Indications for immunohistochemical staining in hepatitis B virus infection.

- To investigate possible cases of HBeAg negative chronic hepatitis B
- To exclude co-existing hepatitis delta virus infection
- To exclude hepatitis B virus infection as a cause of lobular hepatitis in an immunosuppressed patient
- To confirm the aetiology of ground glass hepatocytes (rare)

staining with and without cytoplasmic staining (Figures 4.8 and 4.9). The latter also correlates with active viral replication. It should be noted that the pattern of HBcAg and HBeAg staining can be used as a means of assessing disease activity, although this is not part of routine clinical practice. There is also no clinical role for in situ hybridization to demonstrate hepatitis B virus DNA. It should be noted that hepatitis B virus DNA can sometimes be identified in the liver in patients who are negative for hepatitis B virus DNA in the serum.

Pathology of the immunotolerant phase

The immunotolerant phase is the early phase of chronic hepatitis B virus infection, when the immune response is inadequate and liver damage is mild. Patients in this phase respond poorly to treatment, and the clinician should be advised to withhold therapy and monitor the patient (see page 8).

The histological features of the immunotolerant phase include:
- large numbers of ground glass hepatocytes; and
- mild fibrous expansion of portal tracts with mild portal and lobular inflammation.

Even at this early stage, large cell dysplasia (change) may be seen.

Pathology of the immunoactive phase

In the immunoactive phase of chronic hepatitis B virus infection, an immune response against the virus leads to significant liver damage. Patients in this phase of the disease are likely to develop progressive liver disease and may benefit from therapy – hence therapy is appropriate at this time.

The histological features include:

- architectural changes ranging from fibrous expansion of portal tracts and necroinflammatory changes (e.g. mild or moderate portal inflammation, interface hepatitis, lobular inflammation); and
- possible large cell dysplasia (change).

Ground glass cells are relatively uncommon. Since immunoactive hepatitis B virus infection with cirrhosis may respond poorly to therapy, it is important to alert the clinician if features of cirrhosis are present.

Figure 4.8
Liver biopsy from a patient with hepatitis B stained immunohisto-chemically with an antibody to HBeAg. The predominantly intranuclear staining is characteristic of relatively inactive disease. The presence of HBeAg also confirms the presence of wild type virus.

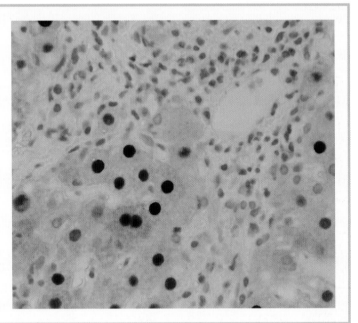

Figure 4.9
Liver biopsy from a patient with HBV stained immunohisto-chemically with an antibody to HBeAg. The widespread intranuclear and cytoplasmic staining indicates active viral replication.

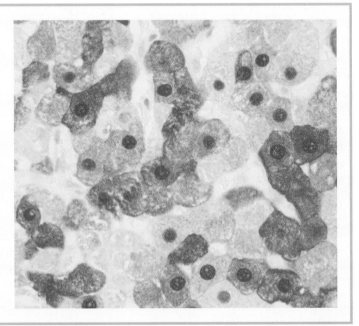

Pathology of the immunosurveillance phase

In the immunosurveillance phase of infection, the virus replicates at very low levels and HBsAg and antibodies against HBeAg are found in the serum. Typically the liver function tests are normal, and a liver biopsy is rarely performed. However, deciding whether a patient has HBeAg-negative chronic hepatitis B (see page 69) or merely hepatitis B surface antigenaemia can be extremely difficult. The viral serology is the same in these two conditions, but in HBeAg-negative chronic hepatitis B liver damage is likely and in hepatitis B surface antigenaemia no injury is expected.

In most patients the diagnosis is straightforward – the liver function tests are normal in patients with isolated hepatitis B surface antigenaemia and abnormal in patients with HBeAg-negative chronic hepatitis B. However, in some patients with HBeAg-negative chronic hepatitis B, the liver function tests fluctuate although they may be normal for many months. To make diagnosis even more difficult, the level of hepatitis B virus DNA in the serum in the two disorders may overlap – typically patients with HBeAg-negative disease have a high level of hepatitis B virus DNA (more than 10^5/ml) and patients with hepatitis B surface antigenaemia have a lower level. However, in HBeAg-negative disease the levels of hepatitis B virus DNA may fluctuate, and some patients with isolated hepatitis B surface antigenaemia have relatively high levels of hepatitis B virus DNA.

Hence, distinguishing between the two can be very difficult, and the liver biopsy may be very helpful in this setting (Table 4.3). The typical histological features in hepatitis B surface antigenaemia include:

- variable degrees of fibrosis;
- mild necroinflammation;
- ground glass hepatocytes; and
- possible large cell dysplasia (change).

Pathology of immunoescape chronic hepatitis B (HBeAg-negative chronic hepatitis B)

In this late phase of infection, mutant hepatitis B virus causes liver damage despite the presence of an immune response directed against the virus. The typical histological features include all the features seen in the immunoactive phase.

In all patients who are HBeAg negative but who have active histological disease the possibility of the patient having developed the mutant virus must be considered. On immunohistochemical staining patients with HBeAg-negative chronic infection show positive staining for HBcAg but are negative for HBeAg. The presence of hepatic HBeAg correlates with circulating wild type virus.

Histological features in immunosuppressed patients

Hepatitis B is occasionally seen in patients with HIV infection and may occur in patients who are immunosuppressed (e.g. as recurrent disease in patients who have had a liver transplant for chronic hepatitis B). Since hepatitis B is an immunopathic virus, in immunosuppressed patients necroinflammatory activity is usually low, although

Table 4.3
A typical liver biopsy report from a patient with hepatitis B virus infection.

Macroscopic appearance
Fragments of brown tissue 2.5 cm in aggregate length
Microscopic appearance
Liver with cirrhotic architecture
There is moderate portal inflammation and interface hepatitis
The bile ducts are normal
There is mild lobular inflammation and ground glass hepatocytes are present
Special stains for iron, alpha-1 antitrypsin bodies and copper-associated protein are negative
There is focal large cell dysplasia
Conclusion
An active cirrhosis with dysplasia due to hepatitis B virus infection
Modified HAI score
Grade – 2+0+1+2=5/18
Stage – 6/6

there is associated active viral replication. On the other hand, in HIV-positive patients improvement in the CD4-positive T-cell counts following highly active anti-retroviral therapy may be associated with a marked increase in liver damage. In some patients who have cleared hepatitis B virus and who are HBeAg-negative, or even HBsAg-negative, immunosuppression may be associated with reactivation of viral infection. The histological picture in these patients is that of lobular (acute) hepatitis. This group of patients includes patients with haematological malignancies being treated with cytotoxic agents. The presence of lobular hepatitis in an immunosup-pressed patient is, therefore, an indication for immunohistochemical staining for hepatitis B virus as well as for cytomegalovirus and other viruses.

A particular form of liver damage was first described in patients who had recurrent hepatitis B virus in their grafted livers – fibrosing cholestatic hepatitis. It is characterized by rapidly progressive liver cell fibrosis associated with bile duct proliferation and liver cell damage. A very similar condition has been reported in a small number of patients with hepatitis B virus infection who have received a renal transplant or who have AIDS. This condition appears to be caused by the exceptionally high viral loads that can be seen in the livers of these patients and the resulting cytopathic liver cell damage.

In immunosuppressed patients, immunohistochemical staining for HBsAg and HBeAg and should always be carried out if there is no other obvious cause for the liver damage seen. This is true both in patients with a lobular hepatitis and in those with fibrosis and bile duct proliferation.

Further reading

Broderick AL, Jonas MM. Hepatitis B in children. *Semin Liver Dis* 2003; **23**: 59–68.

Carmen W, Jacyna M, Hadziyannis S et al. Mutation preventing formation of e antigen in patients with chronic HBV infection. *Lancet* 1989; **2**: 588–91.

Chisari FV, Ferrari C. Hepatitis B virus immunopathogenesis. *Annu Rev Immunol* 1995; **13**: 29–60.

Fattovich G. Natural history and prognosis of hepatitis B. *Semin Liver Dis* 2003; **23**: 47–58.

Ganem D. The molecular biology of the hepatitis B virus. *Annu Rev Biochem* 1987; **56**: 651–93.

Geller SA. Hepatitis B and hepatitis C. *Clin Liver Dis* 2002; **6**: 317–34.

Liaw Y, Chu C, Su I, Huang M, Lin D, Chang C. Clinical and histological events preceeding hepatitis B e antigen seroconversion in chronic Type B hepatitis. *Gastroenterology* 1983; **84**: 216–19.

Lok A, Lai C. Acute exacerbations in Chinese patients with chronic hepatitis B virus infection: incidence, predisposing factors and etiology. *J Hepatol* 1990; **10**: 29–34.

Yeo W, Zee B, Zhong S et al. Comprehensive analysis of risk factors associating with Hepatitis B virus (HBV) reactivation in cancer patients undergoing cytotoxic chemotherapy. *Br J Cancer.* 2004; **90**: 1306–11.

Mills CT, Lee E, Perrillo R. Relationship between histologic, aminotransferase levels, and viral replication in chronic hepatitis B. *Gastroenterology* 1990; **99**: 519–24.

Nakamoto Y, Kaneko S. Mechanisms of viral hepatitis induced liver injury. *Curr Mol Med* 2003; **3**: 537–44.

Perrillo RP, Brunt EM. Hepatic histologic and immunohistochemical changes in chronic hepatitis B after prolonged clearance of hepatitis B e antigen and hepatitis B surface antigen. *Ann Intern Med* 1991; **115**: 113–15.

Poynard T, Lai CL, Ratziu V, Yuen MF, Poynard T. Viral hepatitis B. *Lancet* 2003; **362**: 2089–94.

Questions

1. Regarding the hepatitis B virus:
   A. The X protein crosses the placenta and induces a state of tolerance
   B. The reverse transcriptase enzyme is similar to the HIV enzyme, and some drugs act in both diseases
   C. Elimination of the cccDNA is required to clear all replicating forms
   D. The surface protein is produced in vast excess
   E. HBeAg is encoded by the same gene that codes for the core protein

2. During chronic hepatitis B virus infection:
   A. The immunotolerant phase is characterized by high levels of virus and severe liver damage
   B. The seroconversion reaction involves loss of HBeAg and the development of antibodies against HBeAg, and it is clinically silent
   C. If HBeAg is not detected in serum, any liver disease that is present cannot be due to hepatitis B virus
   D. The severity of the liver damage is not necessarily dependent on the levels of viral replication
   E. Adult infection usually leads to an acute infection

3. In a liver biopsy from a patient with chronic hepatitis B:
   A. The ground glass hepatocytes are a unique feature of chronic hepatitis B virus infection
   B. Immunohistochemical staining is of no value
   C. Interface hepatitis (piecemeal necrosis) indicates autoimmune liver disease
   D. Lymphocytes are typically associated with hepatocytes since the liver disease is due to immune-mediated destruction of infected cells
   E. Dysplastic hepatocytes may indicate that the patient has an increased risk of developing liver cell cancer

4. The following may help to distinguish between the immunosurveillance phase of hepatitis B (hepatitis B surface antigenaemia) and HBeAg-negative chronic hepatitis B:
   A. Serum HBV DNA levels
   B. Titre of IgM anticore antibodies
   C. Immunohistochemistry of a liver biopsy specimen
   D. Titre of HBsAg
   E. Liver function tests

Answers

Question 1

A. False – the HBeAg behaves in this way
B. True
C. True
D. True
E. True

Question 2

A. False – during the immunotolerant phase the virus replicates at high levels but the absence of an immune response ensures that the liver damage is mild
B. False – this seroconversion reaction is usually associated with an increase in the severity of the hepatitis
C. False – HBeAg-negative chronic hepatitis B is associated with significant liver injury
D. True
E. True

Question 3

A. False – a number of other conditions can also give rise to ground glass cells
B. False – immunohistochemistry may aid in distinguishing between the immuno-surveillance phase of chronic hepatitis B and the HBeAg-negative chronic hepatitis B
C. False – it may be seen in a number of chronic liver diseases including viral hepatitis and primary biliary cirrhosis
D. True
E. True

Question 4

A. True
B. True
C. True
D. False
E. True

Management of chronic hepatitis B virus infection

5

The diagnosis and management of chronic hepatitis B virus infection is based on an understanding of its natural history, which has been discussed in Chapter 4.

Diagnosis

Patients with chronic hepatitis B virus infection are typically referred when a virology laboratory reports the presence of HBsAg in serum. The full hepatitis B virological profile of such patients should be assessed for:

- the HBeAg status and antibodies against HBeAg;
- the HBcAb status; and
- liver function tests.

The results of the investigations should be reviewed to determine both the nature and the phase of the infection.

The first step is to determine whether the infection is acute or chronic. A history of recent exposure to the virus (via sexual or other contact) with jaundice, malaise and markedly abnormal liver function tests (transaminase levels over 500 IU/ml) is suggestive of an acute infection, and this is usually confirmed by the finding of a high titre of IgM antibodies to the HBcAg (IgM HBcAb). Although the presence of IgM HBcAb is usually regarded as proof of an acute infection, these antibodies may also develop during activation of a chronic infection (i.e. during conversion from the immunotolerant to the immunoactive phase), and therefore the presence of IgM antibodies should be regarded as strongly suggestive of an acute infection and not as proof of recent infection. During acute hepatitis B virus infection, the virological markers of infection change rapidly and thus all or no antigens may be present (HBsAg and HBeAg) and antibodies against hepatitis B virus may or may not be identified.

Once acute infection has been excluded, the phase of the hepatitis B virus infection should be determined by examining the HBeAg status. If HBeAg is detected in serum then the patient is viraemic and the liver function tests should be analyzed.

If the liver function tests are normal or near normal, the patient is most likely to be in the immunotolerant phase of the disease, and therapy is normally withheld until there is evidence of activity. Measurement of the level of viraemia in these patients is usually of little diagnostic value – if measured, the serum hepatitis B virus DNA concentration is likely to be high (often around 10^7–10^9 copies/ml). A liver biopsy at this stage is helpful to exclude cirrhosis and to confirm the phase of the disease.

If the liver function tests are abnormal then immunoactive disease is likely. A liver biopsy should be taken to confirm the diagnosis and to exclude cirrhosis. Early therapy should be considered. Once again, assessment of the viral load is unlikely to be of diagnostic value but knowledge of the pretreatment viral load is helpful if therapy with a reverse transcriptase inhibitor is planned. High hepatitis B virus DNA levels are to be expected.

Patients who are HBeAg-negative should be assessed to determine whether there is residual virus and disease activity (HBeAg-negative disease) or whether the patient simply has persisting hepatitis B virus surface antigenaemia. As discussed in Chapter 4, it can be surprisingly difficult to distinguish between these two forms of disease. The liver function tests provide the most diagnostic information in this setting – if they are normal, persisting hepatitis B virus surface antigenaemia is probable and the patient is less likely to develop further disease. If the hepatitis B virus DNA level is measured directly it is found to be low or undetectable (usually less than 10^4 copies/ml).

Patients with persisting hepatitis B virus surface antigenaemia are often discharged from further follow-up. In our view it is prudent to keep these patients under distant review, and we monitor all such patients every year to identify late disease reactivation.

Patients with HBeAg-negative chronic hepatitis B are usually identified by the liver function tests. If the liver function tests are abnormal the most likely diagnosis is the presence of mutant hepatitis B virus that does not produce HBeAg (HBeAg-negative disease). This diagnosis should be confirmed by measuring the hepatitis B virus DNA levels, which will be elevated (more than 10^5 copies/ml), and alternative diagnoses (e.g. hepatitis delta virus superinfection, drug reactions) should be considered and excluded by a careful history and a liver biopsy. Some patients with HBeAg-negative chronic hepatitis B have relapsing–remitting disease in which the liver function tests are normal for long periods of time but occasionally relapse with an acute hepatitis-like picture. During the quiescent period the hepatitis B virus DNA levels may be very low but they are usually elevated just before a flare of the disease. This unusual form of chronic hepatitis B can usually be identified by careful observation over a period of several months but, because the hepatitic flares (when the liver function tests are elevated and the hepatitis B virus DNA levels are raised) may be transient, identification can be difficult. In the hepatitic flares that are common in HBeAg-negative chronic hepatitis B, the IgM HBcAb titre is often raised, and this increase may persist for some months. This has led some to suggest that detection of high levels of IgM HBcAb should be used routinely to diagnose HBeAg-negative chronic hepatitis B, but the sensitivity and specificity of this approach have not been rigorously tested.

The HBeAg-negative form of hepatitis B was first identified by genome sequencing of the hepatitis B virus precore region in patients with active liver disease and undetectable HBeAg. A single nucleotide substitution at position 1896 was found in these patients and has since been reported in a high proportion of patients with HBeAg-negative disease. It is tempting to use the identification of this mutation as a diagnostic tool for the HBeAg-negative form of hepatitis B, and many groups have used viral sequencing in an effort to predict who will go on to develop HBeAg-negative disease. These studies have shown that a high proportion of patients with 'normal' virus (i.e. HBeAg-positive chronic hepatitis B) carry the mutant virus and many of them eventually eliminate all traces of the virus. Hence the presence of the mutant

virus cannot be used to predict who will develop HBeAg-negative disease. In patients who have HBeAg-negative chronic hepatitis B, sequencing of the precore region may reveal the presence of the common 1896 pre-core mutation. However, many patients develop other mutations that lead to the same phenotype and thus routine sequencing of the genome of hepatitis B is of no diagnostic or therapeutic value.

An algorithm for the diagnosis of hepatitis B is shown in Figure 5.1. One of the most difficult problems in the diagnosis of chronic hepatitis B is distinguishing between hepatitis B surface antigenaemia and HBeAg-negative chronic hepatitis B. Many patients who are HBsAg-positive and HBeAg-negative are referred for advice and therapy, and the majority are in the immunosurveillance phase of the disease that does not require therapy. A minority have HBeAg-negative disease but this rare condition can only be diagnosed by regular review over many months, with at least one liver biopsy. The clinician is faced with the problem of how to investigate the patient appropriately while avoiding unnecessary investigations.

Since HBeAg-negative disease is now quite common, particularly in patients over the age of 40 intensive monitoring is appropriate in all patients who are HBsAg positive. We review such patients every 3 months for the first year and, if the liver function tests become abnormal during this time, we perform hepatitis B virus DNA assays and a liver biopsy. If the liver function tests remain normal during this year of intensive monitoring, we review the patient on an annual basis.

Figure 5.1
Diagnostic algorithm for patients with chronic hepatitis B infection.

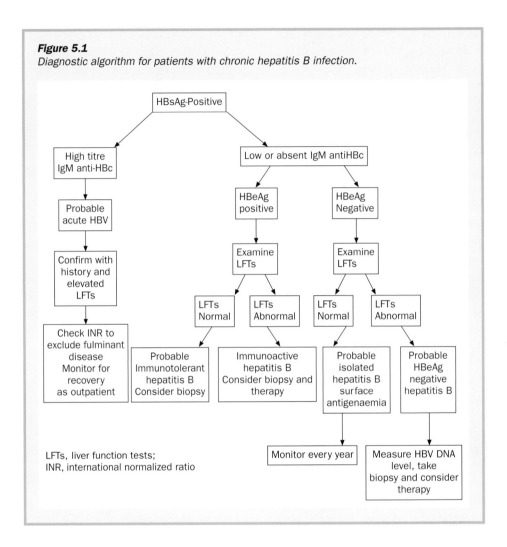

LFTs, liver function tests;
INR, international normalized ratio

Management of the patient with chronic hepatitis B virus infection

Prevention of transmission

All patients who have evidence of ongoing hepatitis B virus infection are at risk of transmitting the virus to others. The risk is greatest in those who are HBeAg-positive or who have high level viraemia (more than 10^5 copies/ml), but even those who are HBeAg-negative with low level viraemia may, albeit rarely, transmit the infection.

All partners and close contacts of patients with HBV infection must be vaccinated to protect them from infection.

The standard hepatitis B vaccine uses HBsAg particles produced in yeast, and the vaccine is well tolerated and safe. The vast majority of vaccinated people respond well and develop antibodies against HBsAg, but a small proportion (5%) do not; in those at high risk of infection (e.g. close contacts of infected patients) it is therefore prudent to check the effectiveness of the vaccination schedule by assessing the antibody response (by measuring the titre of antibodies against HBsAg) 6 months after the last injection. A titre of more than 10 IU/ml is protective but most authorities recommend that the antibody titre should be maintained at more than 100 IU/ml (see Chapter 1 for further discussion of the value of monitoring the antibody response).

For high risk people who have shown a partial response to the vaccine (i.e. those who have developed low antibody titres), further injections of the standard vaccine are recommended, but for those who have shown no response at all, further innoculations are unlikely to be of benefit. For such vaccine 'non-responders' there is currently no effective vaccine although new modified vaccines are being developed and may be available in the future.

Active vaccination against hepatitis B virus is effective but the antibodies are produced only a few months after inoculation. For unprotected people who have been exposed to hepatitis B virus, passive vaccination with anti-hepatitis B serum (HBIg) should be considered (Table 5.1). This expensive prophylaxis should be reserved for those who have had significant contact with the virus and are not already protected by vaccination (e.g. medical personnel exposed to a needle stick injury who have not responded to the standard vaccine). HBIg is widely used for children born to HBeAg-positive mothers; it is given to the newborn baby immediately after birth in association with active vaccination, usually in the contralateral arm.

Although the current vaccines against hepatitis B virus protect most people from infection, a tiny proportion of vaccinated people become infected with hepatitis B virus despite the presence of antibodies against the standard vaccine. Analysis of the virus in these people shows that they are usually infected with a mutant virus (a 'vaccine-escape' mutant) that changes the structure of the envelope protein such that antibodies against the vaccine do not neutralize the viruses. These mutant strains of hepatitis B are rare but there is concern that the increasing use of current vaccines will lead to the widespread development of vaccine-resistant strains.

Table 5.1
Vaccination schedules for hepatitis B.[a]

| Standard vaccination: |
| 0   Month 1   Month 6 |
| Accelerated vaccination: |
| 0   Month 1   Month 2   Month 12 |

[a]The vaccine should be administered by intramuscular injection into the deltoid muscle (the vaccine is less effective when administered into the buttock).

Therapy for patients with chronic hepatitis B virus infection

All patients with chronic hepatitis B virus infection should receive appropriate counselling about:

- infectivity;
- viral transmission; and
- possible therapeutic interventions.

Therapeutic options

The goal of therapy for patients with chronic HBV infection is to prolong life by reducing hepatic inflammation and fibrosis in the long term. Unfortunately most of the current treatment options have only been available for a short time and the effects of the different therapies on survival have not been adequately assessed. Therefore management of chronic HBV infection is based on surrogate markers of disease activity and there is a hierarchy of response to therapy with different treatment end-points being more or less desirable. The most desirable therapeutic end-point is loss of all markers of viral replication and the development of antibodies against both HBeAg and HBsAg. This goal is rarely achieved and most treatment regimens focus on suppressing viral replication and normalizing liver function tests for as long as possible. For patients who have HBeAg-positive disease, loss of HBeAg and the development of anti-HBe antibodies ('seroconversion') is usually associated with prolonged remission of disease activity and is highly desirable. However, the possibility of disease reactivation and the development of

HBeAg negative chronic hepatitis B infection prevents this end-point being regarded as curative. In patients who do not eliminate HBeAg the aim of therapy is to normalize the liver function tests, reduce viraemia and improve liver histology for as long as possible. For patients who have HBeAg-negative chronic hepatitis B, HBeAg seroconversion is clearly an unattainable goal and the focus of therapy should be on reducing viraemia and improving liver histology in the long term. These therapeutic goals are outlined in Table 5.2.

There are two broad approaches to therapy in patients with chronic hepatitis B virus infection:

- immunostimulation with interferon; and
- prolonged suppression of viral replication with a reverse transcriptase (polymerase – POL) inhibitor.

Here we will review the available therapies before discussing their use in the different phases of the disease.

Interferon therapy in chronic HBV infection

Interferon therapy was introduced for patients with chronic HBeAg-positive hepatitis B in the late 1980s and most treatment regimens involve a 4–6 month course of high dose interferon monotherapy – 5–9 MIU three times a week. Interferon is a potent antiviral cytokine and within a few days of commencing therapy there is a marked decrease in viraemia and an improvement in liver function tests. In a proportion of patients viral suppression is followed by the development of an enhanced immune response against the virus that is

Table 5.2
Therapeutic goals for patients with chronic hepatitis B virus infection.

Hierarchy of response		
All patients	1	Development of antiHBs antibodies
	2	Loss of HBsAg
Patients who are HBeAg positive	3	Development of anti-HBe antibodies
	4	Loss of HBeAg
	5	Histological improvement
	6	Prolonged normalization of liver function tests associated with reduction in circulating viraemia
Patients who are HBeAg negative	3	Histological improvement
	4	Prolonged normalization of liver function tests associated with reduction in circulating viraemia

usually associated with a transient increase in hepatocyte damage and an increase in serum transaminases – the so-called 'seroconversion hepatitis', that typically develops some 12 weeks after the initiation of treatment. In the majority of patients who develop this seroconversion reaction antibodies against HBeAg develop and when the interferon therapy is discontinued high level viral replication does not return and the patient enters the immunosurveillance phase of the disease. In patients who do not develop antibodies against HBeAg treatment cessation is invariably associated with the return of high level viral replication and liver damage. In a small proportion of patients receiving interferon therapy HBeAg seroconversion is followed by the loss of HBsAg and the development of antibodies against this protein. This is usually associated with long-term, probably lifelong, disease remission.

For patients with HBeAg negative disease interferon therapy clearly can not induce a seroconversion reaction and therapy is normally given for one or more years. In the majority of patients treatment leads to a reduction in viraemia and improvement in liver histology but once therapy is withdrawn the viraemia and associated liver damage usually recur, although a proportion of patients do derive long-term benefit in terms of reduced liver inflammation for many months after treatment cessation. Since interferon is associated with numerous side effects prolonged therapy (i.e. for more than 2 years) is likely to be poorly tolerated.

Trials of PEG-IFNα2a (40 KD) in patients with chronic HBV infection are currently under way. Since this pegylated interferon is easier to use and associated with fewer side effects than conventional interferon this regimen is likely to prove popular with patients and results of early clinical trials indicate that pegylated interferons may be significantly more effective both in HBeAg positive and HBeAg negative disease. Similarly trials of the PEG-IFNα2b (12KD) in HBeAg positive disease are in progress and this long lasting IFN also appears to be superior to conventional IFN.

Reverse transcriptase inhibitors

Two reverse transcriptase inhibitors (lamivudine and adefovir) are currently licensed for the therapy of patients with chronic hepatitis B virus infection but alternative drugs are currently undergoing clinical trials. All of the reverse transcriptase inhibitors suppress viral replication and, for patients with HBeAg-positive disease prolonged suppression of viral replication is often associated with the development of an immune response against the virus that leads to an HBeAg seroconversion reaction.

Lamivudine is a nucleoside analogue that is a potent reverse transcriptase inhibitor. It successfully suppresses hepatitis B virus replication in the medium term. The drug is extremely well tolerated with a very good safety profile but prolonged therapy leads to the development of lamivudine-resistant mutations. These occur with a frequency of around 15% per year and usually involve mutations in the YMDD motif within the polymerase protein. The development of these mutations is associated with a return of viraemia and an increase in liver inflammation. However, lamivudine-resistant mutant viruses are usually, but not always, associated with impaired viral replication so that when lamivudine resistance develops both the viral load and liver inflammation are reduced when compared to the values

before treatment initiation. In some patients, lamivudine resistance may be associated with seroconversion reactions and in many patients the development of lamivudine resistance is associated with histological regression in the short term. However, seroconversion rates in patients with lamivudine-resistant infections are reduced when compared with the response rates in patients with lamivudine-sensitive virus and the development of lamivudine resistance may be associated with transient increases in serum transaminases (hepatic flares) as high level viral replication recurs. In patients with cirrhosis and, very occasionally in patients who do not have cirrhosis, these flares may lead to hepatic decompensation and even death, and close monitoring is therefore required.

> *Lamivudine is active against HIV replication and high dose lamivudine therapy is a widely used component of anti-HIV treatment regimens. The low dose lamivudine monotherapy used to treat hepatitis B rapidly induces resistance in HIV and therefore all patients with hepatitis B who require lamivudine should be tested for HIV BEFORE therapy is instituted.*

Hence lamivudine is a safe, well tolerated antiviral agent that effectively suppresses viral replication in the medium term and often induces HBeAg seroconversion reactions. Its long-term efficacy is restricted by the development of resistance mutations that may be associated with disease progression or serious adverse events.

Adefovir

Adefovir depivoxil is a nucleotide analogue that effectively suppresses hepatitis B virus replication. Clinical trials with adefovir over 3 years have shown that the drug at a dose of 10 mg/day has an excellent safety profile and induces resistant mutations at a very low rate – less than 2% per year. Of great importance is that the drug is active against the common lamivudine-resistant mutants (the YMDD mutant) and therefore can be used to treat patients who have experienced relapse while receiving lamivudine. Although adefovir is a very potent inhibitor of the HBV polymerase the decrease in HBV DNA that occurs when this agent is commenced is sometimes rather slow and some patients need treatment for many months before the viral load decreases to undetectable levels.

Therapy in patients with HBeAg-positive chronic hepatitis B

Immunotolerant phase

During the early phase of chronic hepatitis B virus infection (the immunotolerant phase with high level viraemia and normal liver function tests), there is no effective immune response against the virus, and immunostimulation with conventional interferon is almost always ineffective and should be avoided. Likewise, therapy with lamivudine leads to suppression of viraemia but, since there is no pre-existing immune response, the virus is not eliminated and there is a high risk of the development of lamivudine-resistant mutants (see page 88). However, recent trials with the PEG-IFNα2a (40KD) show that a proportion of patients with immunotolerant hepatitis B do seroconvert when treated for 6 months and the low mutation rates seen with adefovir suggest that this drug may have a role to play in patients in this phase of the disease. However, since liver damage during the immunotolerant phase of chronic hepatitis B is usually minimal it is more appropriate to defer therapy until the disease moves into the immunoactive phase when therapy has a much greater chance of success. A liver biopsy is important to exclude significant disease and patients with evidence of fibrosis or significant inflammation should receive therapy. Patients with normal liver function tests and minimal disease on a liver biopsy should be advised that their liver is not being damaged, and liver function tests should be monitored every 6 months. Any increase in the transaminase level should prompt an increase in the intensity of monitoring and, if the increase in liver inflammation (i.e. increased alanine aminotransferase) is maintained for more than 3 months, it is likely that the disease has moved into the second phase, the immunoactive phase.

> *Management of the immunotolerant phase of hepatitis B virus infection involves a liver biopsy to exclude significant disease and close observation. Therapy is best avoided as response rates are low but treatment with a pegylated interferon or adefovir may be considered.*

of at least 12 months with low-dose interferon alfa (3–5 MIU three times a week) has been shown to induce a sustained response (i.e. no recurrence of disease or viraemia after 12 months) in no more than 20% of treated patients. Trials with the PEG-IFNα2a (40KD) show that after 48 weeks of therapy up to 36% of patients have a sustained response (defined as normal LFTs and low level viraemia) that persists for at least 24 weeks off therapy. A small proportion of patients receiving the PEG-IFNα2a (40KD) develop antibodies against surface antigen and therefore therapy with this drug may be regarded as 'curative' in 4% and 'beneficial in the medium term' in a further 30–40%.

Treatment of HBeAg-negative chronic hepatitis B with lamivudine is beneficial in the short term – the viraemia declines and the liver function tests improve. However, if the therapy is discontinued after 1 year the virus almost invariably recurs. Prolonged therapy leads to the development of lamivudine resistance and return of viraemia, and after 3 years of therapy up to 50% of treated patients have developed lamivudine-resistant mutants. In these patients, in whom an immunological viral clearance is not possible, the development of lamivudine resistance is not associated with eventual viral clearance, and the emergence of resistant viral strains may be associated with further progression of the liver damage.

Adefovir therapy is effective in patients with HBeAg negative chronic HBV and, like lamivudine, viral replication is suppressed and liver function tests and liver

histology improve in the short term. However, prolonged therapy with adefovir is rarely associated with the development of drug-resistant mutants and current data indicates that the majority of patients will derive benefit from therapy for at least 3 years.

In patients with HBeAg-negative chronic infection combination therapy with pegylated interferon and lamivudine conveys no benefits over the first 12 months but trials with multiple nucleos(t)ide analogues have not yet been performed. It is likely that combination therapy with lamivudine and adefovir will prove to be effective in reducing the rate of development of mutations but it is not yet clear whether this will be cost effective when compared to therapy with adefovir alone.

At present, there is no consensus on the most effective therapy for HBeAg-negative chronic hepatitis B but data from ongoing and future clinical trials seem likely to address the question of the most efficacious, cost-effective treatment regimen. For patients who are stable with mild fibrosis, therapy may best be deferred until more information is available. For patients with advancing fibrosis who are at risk of developing cirrhosis, the options include long-term pegylated interferon therapy or prolonged therapy with a nucleos(t)ide analogue. At present, the authors offer pegylated interferon or lamivudine to patients with HBeAg-negative disease who do not have cirrhosis, and for those who elect to undergo therapy with lamivudine we introduce adefovir monotherapy when resistance eventually does develop.

Further reading

De Franchis R et al. EASL International Consensus Conference on Hepatitis B. *J Hepatol* 2003; **39**: S3–S25.

Dienstag JL, Schiff ER, Wright TL et al. Lamivudine as initial treatment for chronic hepatitis B in the United States. *N Engl J Med* 1999; **341**: 1256–63.

Keefe EB et al. A treatment algorithm for the management of chronic hepatitis B virus infection in the United States. *Clin Gastroenterol Hepatol* 2004; **2**: 87–106.

Lavanchy D. Hepatitis B virus epidemiology, disease burden, treatment, and current and emerging and control measures: a review. *J Viral Hepat* 2004; **11**: 97–107.

Marcellin P et al. Peginterferon alfa 2a alone, lamivudine alone and the two in combination in patients with HBeAg – negative chronic hepatitis B. *N Engl J Med* 2004; **16**: 1206–17.

Papatheodoridis GV, Hadziyannis SJ. Diagnosis and management of pre-core mutant chronic hepatitis B. *J Viral Hep* 2001; **8:** 311–21.

Questions

1. In patients with HBeAg-positive chronic hepatitis B who are receiving interferon based therapy:
    A. An increase in the serum transaminase level indicates that therapy is not working
    B. Treatment should be given indefinitely
    C. The platelet count may decrease
    D. Cirrhosis may deteriorate
    E. Anaemia is a common complication

2. Lamivudine therapy for chronic hepatitis B:
    A. Is given by injection
    B. Leads to seroconversion in 75% of patients after 1 year
    C. May induce mutations in the polymerase protein
    D. May synergize with interferon
    E. Is best given during the immunoactive phase

3. HBeAg-negative chronic hepatitis B:
    A. Is always benign
    B. Should be treated with 3 months of interferon
    C. May be treated for several years with adefovir with a low incidence of resistant mutations
    D. May be associated with an increase in the IgM anti-HBcAg titre
    E. Is always resistant to lamivudine

4. Therapy for chronic hepatitis B:
    A. Should be given when the disease is quiescent
    B. May be most effective when the liver function tests are abnormal
    C. Always requires multiple drugs
    D. May cause a transient increase in the severity of the hepatitis
    E. May generate lamivudine-resistant mutants

Answers

Question 1

A. False – an increase in the serum transaminases often indicates that an immune response is developing that may lead to a seroconversion
B. False – therapy for 3–6 months is adequate
C. True
D. True
E. False

Question 2

A. False – it is an oral therapy
B. False
C. True
D. False
E. True

Question 3

A. False
B. False – at least 12 months interferon therapy is required
C. True
D. True
E. False

Question 4

A. False
B. True
C. False
D. True
E. True

Combined infections

6

Simultaneous infection with more than one virus is unusual, probably because the host defences are activated by the first virus and are then primed and ready to prevent further infections. As discussed in Chapter 1, hepatotropic viruses are able to avoid the host defence systems and this allows infection with multiple different viruses. Even so, patients with more than one infection are uncommon and, in general, the presence of more than one pathogen accelerates disease progression.

Hepatitis delta virus

The hepatitis delta virus is a unique human pathogen that needs the hepatitis B virus to infect cells and cause disease. Hepatitis delta virus is unable to cause infection on its own because it lacks an envelope protein, and the virus requires the surface antigen of the hepatitis B virus in order to propagate itself.

The virus and its replication

The hepatitis delta virus consists of a circular RNA genome that encodes a single protein, the delta antigen. The virus replicates in an unusual fashion that is similar to the process used by plant viroids. The viral RNA is duplicated in a 'rolling circle' mechanism in which antigenomic RNA is produced in a long chain; the long chain of multiple, joined viral genomes is then cleaved by a ribozyme. Ribozymes are enzymes that are formed by loops of RNA and are able to

Figure 6.1
Liver biopsy from a patient with chronic HBV who developed a flare up of his disease due to superinfection with hepatitis delta virus. Histologically this was characterized by active lobular inflammation.

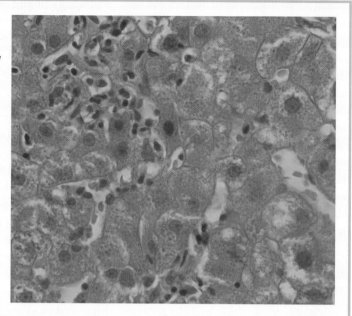

Figure 6.2
Same liver biopsy as in Figure 6.1 stained with an antibody to hepatitis delta virus. The positive nuclear staining illustrated is sensitive and specific confirmation of active infection by hepatitis delta virus.

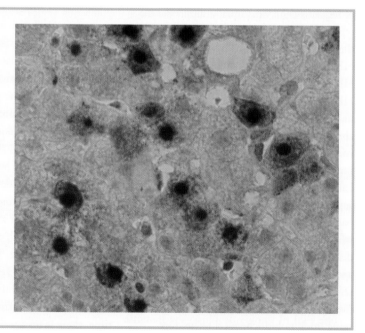

available antibody to the hepatitis delta antigen. In liver transplant patients, hepatitis delta virus antigen can be demonstrated in the absence of hepatitis B. The associated liver damage in these circumstances is very mild.

Management of chronic hepatitis delta virus infection

Although there is no vaccine against hepatitis delta virus itself, the virus depends on the presence of hepatitis B virus for its replication; therefore preventing infection with hepatitis B also protects against the hepatitis delta agent. Hence contacts and partners of patients with chronic hepatitis delta should be vaccinated against hepatitis B.

A typical liver biopsy report from a patient with hepatitis B virus infection and superimposed hepatitis delta virus infection is shown in Table 6.1.

Patients infected with hepatitis delta virus are at high risk of developing progressive liver disease. It is therefore unfortunate that there is at present no proven, effective therapy for patients with this disease. Short courses of interferon have been tried in patients with chronic hepatitis delta but they are usually

Table 6.1
A typical liver biopsy report from a patient with hepatitis B virus infection and superimposed hepatitis delta virus infection.

Macroscopic appearance
A core of brown tissue 2.9 cm in length

Microscopic appearance
Liver with widespread fibrous expansion of portal tracts
There is mild portal inflammation and interface hepatitis but there is marked lobular inflammation with prominent acidophilic degeneration of hepatocytes
The bile ducts are normal
No ground glass cells are present
Special stains for iron, alpha-1-anti-trypsin bodies and copper-associated protein are negative
There is no dysplasia

Immunohistochemical staining
5% of cells show nuclear ± cytoplasmic staining for delta antigen
There is focal cytoplasmic staining for HBsAg; staining for HBcAg is negative

Conclusion
An active chronic hepatitis due to hepatitis delta virus infection in a patient with hepatitis B

Modified HAI score
Grade – 1+0+3+1=5/18
Stage – 2/6

unsuccessful and the pegylated interferons have not been assessed in this setting. Lamivudine is ineffective and the efficacy of the recently developed reverse transcriptase inhibitors that are more potent than lamivudine have not been assessed in patients with delta virus. Results with these agents are awaited with interest.

To date the only successful therapy for delta virus infection is prolonged therapy with high doses of conventional interferon (up to 5–10 MIU given daily). This punishing schedule needs to be maintained for at least 2 years and very often treatment discontinuation is associated with return of viraemia and liver damage that requires a further course of therapy. It is to be hoped that clinical trials with the pegylated interferons will show that these agents are more effective than the conventional interferons.

Co-infection with other viruses

Co-infection, either with several hepatotropic viruses or with a hepatotropic virus and HIV, is fortunately rare; however, when it does occur interactions between the different viruses alter both the natural history of the disease and the treatment.

Hepatitis B virus and hepatitis C virus co-infection

Since these two viruses are both blood-borne pathogens, it would be expected that co-infection should be quite common. However, this does not appear to be the case, and co-infection is much less prevalent than predicted. When co-infection is found, it is usually associated with a rapidly progressive disease that leads to cirrhosis within a few years.

The presence of both hepatitis B virus and hepatitis C virus usually leads to inhibition of the replication of one of them. Thus, patients tend to have high levels of hepatitis C viraemia with low levels of hepatitis B virus DNA and undetectable HBeAg, or they tend to be HBeAg-positive with high levels of hepatitis B virus DNA and low levels of hepatitis C virus RNA. In some patients the dominant virus may change with time, and such patients may therefore have dominant hepatitis B on one occasion and dominant hepatitis C on another.

Co-infection with hepatitis B and hepatitis C is very difficult to treat. Conventional therapeutic regimens of pegylated interferon–ribavirin or lamivudine are rarely successful. Logically these patients should benefit from therapy with interferon plus ribavirin plus lamivudine, but the safety and efficacy of this approach has never been tested and further clinical studies are urgently required in this group of patients.

Although co-infection with hepatitis B virus and hepatitis C virus is uncommon, a number of patients with active hepatitis C have evidence of past exposure to hepatitis B virus (i.e. they have antibodies against the viral proteins, such as anti-hepatitis B virus core antibodies). It is becoming clear that these patients tend to have a diminished response to therapy for their chronic hepatitis C, although the reasons for this are not yet clear.

HIV and hepatitis C virus co-infection

In the past, HIV and hepatitis C virus co-infection was of little hepatological importance as, sadly, patients died of HIV-related immunosuppression long before liver damage developed. Effective anti-retroviral therapy (Highly Active Anti-Retroviral Therapy, HAART) has led to a reappraisal of the significance of co-infection and it is now clear that infection with HIV and hepatitis C virus leads to an increase in the severity of both infections: the natural history of chronic hepatitis C infection is accelerated in patients who are co-infected and progression to cirrhosis is both more rapid and more common. This increase in the severity of liver disease in co-infected patients has led to liver disease becoming one of the most common causes of death in HIV-positive patients in the USA.

In addition to the deleterious effects of HIV on hepatitis C, it is now believed that hepatitis C may accelerate the progression of HIV infection and co-infected patients have evidence of more significant lymphocyte functional abnormalities than patients who are infected only with HIV. Thus co-infection with both hepatitis C and HIV accelerates the progression of both viral infections.

Treatment of patients with HIV–hepatitis C co-infection

Therapy for patients with both HIV and HCV infection is difficult. Concurrent management of two different diseases presents particular challenges and many patients who are co-infected have co-morbid factors (such as depression) that increase the difficulties associated with treatment. The problems of managing these patients are compounded by the rapidly progressive liver disease that is common in co-infected patients and the reduced response rates that are seen in these patients when they are treated with conventional interferons and ribavirins.

Recent clinical trials have clarified the role of combination therapy with pegylated interferon and ribavirin in patients who are co-infected with HCV and HIV. Two large-scale independent clinical trials have recently been completed and Tables 6.2 and 6.3 summarize the results along with the major differences between the two studies.

It is important to recognize that although both of these multicentre clinical trials used low dose ribavirin (800 mg) because of concerns regarding possible interactions with anti-retroviral agents, the trials were different in design and studied different patient populations. Both trials included patients who were or were not taking anti-retroviral medication, but patients with very advanced HIV were excluded. The studies showed that hepatitis C can be eliminated in patients who are co-infected with HIV although the response rates are a little reduced when compared with those seen in patients who are not co-infected. The clinical trials with pegylated interferons and ribavirin in patients who are co-infected with hepatitis C and HIV suggested that therapy was, in general, well tolerated and the incidence of interferon and ribavirin related side effects was not dramatically different from that seen in patients who had isolated chronic

Although ddI therapy must not be combined with ribavirin studies in patients included in the recent clinical trial involving PEG-IFNα2a (40KD) and ribavirin show that intracellular levels of lamivudine (3TC), stavudine (d4T) and zidovudine (AZT) did not change throughout the HCV treatment period so these drugs may be safely combined with ribavirin, although careful monitoring remains essential as dramatic changes in haemoglobin levels and liver function tests are occasionally seen in co-infected patients.

During therapy for co-infection with HCV and HIV the absolute CD4 count often falls. However, the percentage CD4 count usually remains satisfactory and infections related to immunosuppression did not present a problem during the recent clinical trials. Hence during therapy for co-infected patients it is important to monitor percentage CD4 counts and not the absolute count.

A particular problem in co-infected patients is the onset of cirrhosis. Patients with HIV/HCV co-infection who have developed decompensated cirrhosis should not be offered therapy with pegylated interferons as the results are very poor and complications are common. Patients with well compensated cirrhosis can be treated but vigilance is required to detect any side effects at an early stage. A number of patients with HIV/HCV co-infection have undergone liver transplantation with success and this option should therefore be considered although the long-term success of transplantation is not yet known in these complex cases.

HIV and hepatitis B virus co-infection

Careful consideration of the natural history of chronic hepatitis B and the role of the immune system in the pathogenesis of this disease enables the likely effects of concomitant HIV infection to be predicted. During the immunotolerant phase of chronic hepatitis B virus infection, when high-level viraemia is associated with a minimal immune response, co-infection with HIV usually has little impact. However, if the HIV-related immunosuppression is severe then the level of hepatitis B viraemia may rise markedly and fibrosing cholestatic hepatitis may develop, although this is rare (see page 77).

For patients with the immunoactive form of chronic hepatitis B (high level hepatitis B viraemia with an inflammatory response and marked liver damage), significant HIV infection may reduce the liver inflammation. As the immune response is impaired by HIV infection, the immune-mediated liver damage tends to subside.

During the immunosurveillance phase of chronic hepatitis B virus infection (HBsAg-positive, HBeAg-negative serology with low-level viraemia), immunosuppression due to HIV infection may lead to a reverse seroconversion. The reduction in the immune response against hepatitis B virus may lead to a reactivation of the disease and emergence of detectable levels of HBeAg. If the immune response is restored by anti-retroviral therapy, the hepatic infection may be brought under control once again – initially the immune response leads to an increase in liver damage but eventually the immune response may lead to the elimination of the HBeAg once again.

Hence co-infection with HIV may significantly modify the effects of the hepatitis B virus, and careful monitoring of both viruses is required to determine the likely cause of the liver disease. It is important to be aware of the hepatotoxic effects of the widely used anti-retroviral drugs – in patients with HIV infection and hepatitis B virus infection, any change in the liver function tests should be fully investigated, and increases in hepatic inflammation should not be ascribed to activation of the hepatitis B unless other possible causes have been excluded; in general marked changes in liver function tests should be investigated by a liver biopsy in these patients. Immunochemistry is very valuable in assessing liver biopsies from this group of patients.

Management of hepatitis B virus and HIV co-infection

Interferon therapy has been tried in HBV–HIV co-infected patients but there are few reports of success and the benefits of the new pegylated interferons in this group of patients are unclear. For patients with active hepatitis B and HIV co-infection, lamivudine is a logical therapeutic choice because it inhibits the replication of both viruses. However, it is important to be aware of the different doses used in the treatment of these infections – patients with HIV infection require high-dose lamivudine whereas patients with chronic hepatitis B virus infection are usually treated with much lower doses. Close collaboration between the hepatologist and the infectious disease physician is required to ensure that these patients are managed appropriately. It is easy to forget the hepatitis B component of the illness when considering drug changes for the HIV infection, and in co-infected patients the lamivudine therapy should not be stopped even if it is no longer required for suppression of HIV replication.

An alternative approach to lamivudine therapy for co-infected patients is to use another anti-retroviral agent that is active against both hepatitis B and HIV. In this regard tenofovir has useful activity against both viruses and, although not licensed for this indication is often used with success in this setting.

Further reading

Farci P. Delta hepatitis: an update. *J Hepatol* 2003; **39**: S212–19.

Greub G, Ledergerber B, Battegay M et al. Clinical progression, survival, and immune recovery during antiretroviral therapy in patients with HIV-1 and hepatitis C virus coinfection: the Swiss HIV Cohort Study. *Lancet* 2000; **356**: 1800–5.

Mathurin P, Thibault V, Kadidja K et al. Replication status and histological features of patients with triple (B, C, D) and dual (B, C) hepatic infections. *J Viral Hepat* 2000; **7**: 15–22.

Torriani FJ et al. PEG interferon alfa-2a plus ribavirin for chronic hepatitis C virus infection in HIV-infected patients. *NEJM* 2004; **351**: 438–50.

Thio CL. Management of chronic hepatitis B in the HIV-infected patient. *AIDS Read* 2004; **14**: 122–9, 133, 136–7.

change. It has been widely used in clinical trials and may be useful in clinical practice since it allows the extent of the hepatic disease to be assessed. Table 8.1 gives the salient features of this scoring system. All patients with cirrhosis should be evaluated for the presence of oesophageal varices (usually by endoscopy) and, if varices are found, primary prophylaxis with propranolol should be commenced and beta-blockers should be given at a dose that reduces the resting pulse rate by 30%. These patients should be considered for entry into ultrasound screening programmes (see page 139).

Management of hepatitis C-related cirrhosis

Patients with cirrhosis induced by chronic hepatitis C do respond to therapy, albeit at a lower rate than patients with lesser degrees of fibrosis. Follow-up studies comparing treated and untreated patients suggest that the rate of development of decompensated disease and the development of liver cell cancer is reduced in patients who have received interferon therapy. This benefit is most marked in patients who have cleared the virus, but even patients who have not responded to therapy by eliminating the virus may have a reduced rate of complications.

These studies indicate that patients with hepatitis C-related cirrhosis may derive considerable benefit from therapy and studies with the pegylated interferons combined with ribavirin indicate that a significant proportion (over 40%) will respond to treatment. For patients with hepatitis C-induced cirrhosis that is well compensated (Child–Pugh grade A)

Table 8.1
The Child–Pugh score.

Points scored	Encephalopathy grade[a]	Bilirubin (μmol/l)	Albumin (g/l)	Prolongation of prothrombin time (sec)
1	–	<25	>35	1–4
2	I, II	25–40	28–35	4–6
3	III, IV	>40	<28	>6

[a]Grading of encephalopathy:
Grade I – confused, altered mood or behaviour, psychometric defects
Grade II – drowsy, inappropriate behaviour
Grade III – stuporous but speaking and obeying simple commands; inarticulate speech, marked confusion
Grade IV – coma

Grade A is a score of 5–6
Grade B is a score of 7–9
Grade C is a score of 10–15

treatment with a pegylated interferon and ribavirin should be offered. Therapy with interferon invariably leads to a decrease in both the platelet count and the white cell count and, in the presence of hypersplenism, may lead to a dangerous decline in these parameters. In patients with well-compensated cirrhosis who have a platelet count of more than 75×10^9 cells/l and a total white cell count of more than 2.5×10^9 cells/l, this rarely causes significant problems, although dose adjustments may be necessary in some patients. In patients with cirrhosis who have platelet counts and white cell counts that are lower than these levels, interferon therapy may lead to a dangerous fall in either the platelet count or the white cell count, and these patients should receive therapy only in centres with experience in the management of this difficult patient group.

In addition to its antiviral and immunomodulatory effects, interferon has antifibrotic properties and may reduce hepatic fibrosis. This has led to suggestions that patients with cirrhosis who have not eliminated the virus after a course of pegylated interferon plus ribavirin should receive long-term maintenance therapy to improve the underlying fibrosis. This approach is currently being prospectively studied in the USA, where the PEG-IFNα2a (40KD) at a dose of 90 μg/week, will be administered for several years to patients with cirrhosis and advanced fibrosis. The outcome of this study is awaited with interest. In the absence of evidence that prolonged interferon therapy is beneficial to patients with hepatitis C-related cirrhosis we do not routinely use this approach at present.

Patients with hepatitis C who develop decompensated cirrhosis (Child–Pugh grade C) should be considered for liver transplantation, and local guidelines about suitability for surgery should be consulted and applied. Studies with interferon-based therapies in such patients (in particular those with ascites) indicate that there is a high incidence of infection (such as spontaneous bacterial peritonitis) and such patients should not therefore be treated except in the context of clinical trials.

Liver transplantation for chronic hepatitis C-related cirrhosis

The management of patients undergoing liver transplantation is complex and is beyond the scope of this book. For patients with chronic hepatitis C who undergo liver transplantation, either for decompensated liver disease or hepatocellular carcinoma, the short-term outlook is very good. As with all patients undergoing transplantation, the risks of surgery are high but over 80% of patients are likely to survive the operation and return home. Unfortunately the hepatitis C virus always infects the new liver and in some patients the disease recurs in an aggressive form. The natural history of hepatitis C after liver transplantation is not yet known but it is becoming clear that there is a significant increase in mortality over the first 10 years. Thus 20% of patients develop cirrhosis within 1 year of transplantation and a small proportion die of hepatitis C-related liver disease within 5 years of transplantation. Among those who survive the first few years, some have persistent viraemia with no significant liver

Figure 9.3
A fragment of a liver cell cancer biopsy with large cells with hyperchromatic nuclei arranged in a trabecular pattern.

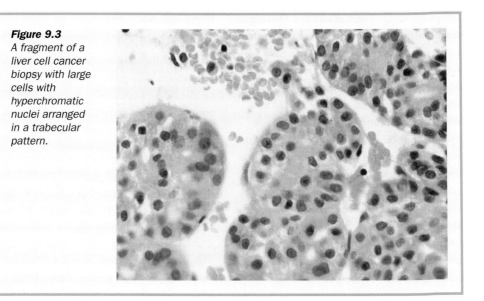

Figure 9.4
The same liver biopsy as in Figure 9.3, showing a marked decrease in reticulin staining compared with normal liver.

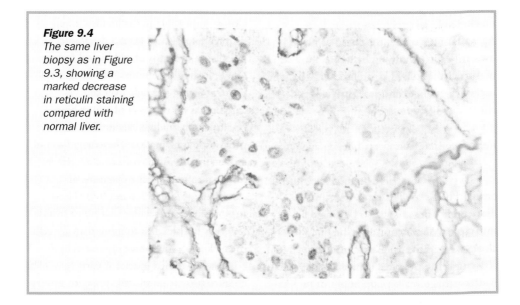

this. However, as is so often the case in histopathology, in the most difficult tumours this feature cannot be relied on for making the diagnosis. Focal fibrosis may be seen in otherwise typical liver cell cancers in areas of necrosis; fibrolamellar carcinomas in which lamellar fibrosis is a clinical feature are not associated with viral hepatitis or cirrhosis.

Another clue that a hepatocyte lesion is malignant is that the endothelial cells lining the sinusoids are CD34-positive; normal endothelial cells lining the hepatic sinusoids are CD34-negative.

A number of other growth patterns may be seen, including:

- a pseudoglandular pattern;
- a solid pattern; and
- a telangiectatic pattern.

Capsular and vascular invasion, which is a very common feature in HCC, may be helpful in making the diagnosis. These variants need to be distinguished especially from metastatic carcinomas. Bile production, while uncommon, is diagnostic of liver cell carcinoma. HCCs are frequently, albeit focally, positive for AFP. Although high serum AFP levels are common in HCC, positive immunohisto-chemical staining is much less commonly seen. Presumably this is because of the rapid rate at which this protein is secreted. Similarly, staining for cytokeratins is sometimes useful in distinguishing liver cell carcinomas from other malignant tumours. If a tumour is negative for cytokeratin 7 it is likely to be a HCC. On the other hand, if a tumour does stain with cytokeratin 7 this does not exclude the possibility that the tumour is a HCC since HCCs, like all other tumours, may show phenotypic differences from their non-neoplastic counterparts. A monoclonal antibody to CD10 may be useful in identifying bile canaliculi in liver cell cancers.

Although HCCs are overwhelmingly the most common malignancy seen in cirrhotic livers, cholangiocarcinomas and metastatic carcinomas should always be considered. It should be noted that adrenal cell carcinomas may also be positive for AFP. While the presence of co-existing cirrhosis makes it very likely that any tumour is an HCC, HCC can arise in non-cirrhotic livers. This is especially true in males living in areas where HCC is very common (e.g. Africa).

Management of the isolated hepatic nodule

Many patients with viral hepatitis develop a nodule within the liver. This is commonly identified during screening for HCC but similar lesions may be found during ultrasound examination for other reasons (e.g. to investigate the upper abdominal pains that are common in patients with chronic hepatitis C). Accurate diagnosis is essential in this instance and the possible causes are listed in Table 9.2. Most experienced ultrasonog-raphers can identify cystic lesions and haemangiomas, and the clinician is left to decide the most appropriate management of a solid hepatic nodule.

If the lesion is an HCC then a liver biopsy may spread the cancer along the needle tract and either on to the skin or throughout the peritoneal cavity. Tumour

Dysplasia

Liver cell dysplasia has been shown to be associated with the development of HCC in patients with chronic hepatitis B and hepatitis C. Most hepatologists agree that the presence of dysplasia on a liver biopsy increases the probability of HCC developing and accordingly they increase the intensity of monitoring or screening appropriately.

There are two forms of liver cell dysplasia:

- large cell dysplasia; and
- small cell dysplasia.

Liver cell dysplasia may been seen in dysplastic nodules or on its own in either cirrhotic or non-cirrhotic livers. Clusters of large cell dysplasia or small cell dysplasia less than 1 mm in diameter have been termed 'dysplastic foci'. When they are larger they are termed 'dysplastic nodules'.

Large cell dysplasia (change)

Large cell dysplasia is characterized by the presence of collections of cells with large nuclei and increased amounts of cytoplasm (Figure 9.5). This means that, despite the size of the nuclei, the nuclear–cytoplasmic ratio is normal. In addition to nuclear enlargement there may be pleomorphism and hyperchromasia as well as multinucleation and increased numbers of nucleoli. This change is recognized more easily if the size of normal hepatocytes, seen elsewhere in the biopsy, is used as an internal control.

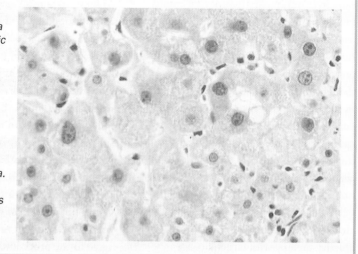

Figure 9.5
Liver biopsy from a patient with chronic hepatitis B. The cells in the top right of the picture contain sheets of hepatocytes with larger nuclei and more abundant cytoplasm. This is characteristic of large cell dysplasia. The nuclear–cytoplasmic ratio is normal.

Large cell dysplasia needs to be distinguished both from the increased nuclear pleomorphism seen in livers with increasing age and from the variability in nuclear size seen as a reactive change in livers with active lobular hepatitis. In addition to the presence of associated clinical and pathological features (i.e. patient's age, presence of active inflammation), another important clue is that the changes seen in liver cell dysplasia involve groups of contiguous hepatocytes rather than scattered cells. Image analysis is not necessary for diagnosing the presence of large cell dysplasia.

The nuclei in large cell dysplasia have been shown to be aneuploid and are associated with chromosomal abnormalities. Despite this, and although large cell dysplasia is associated with a four- to fivefold increased risk of co-existing HCC or of

developing such a tumour, the dysplastic cells are not premalignant. In other words, they are a marker for the development of large cell cancer but are not actually the precursor lesion. Cell kinetic studies indicate that the proliferative rate of these cells is in fact decreased. It is for this reason that some authors prefer the term large cell change. Nevertheless, the presence of large cell dysplasia, especially in patients with chronic hepatitis B, is taken as an indication that a patient needs careful follow-up with serum AFP and liver ultrasound.

Small cell dysplasia (change)

In small cell dysplasia (Figure 9.6), although the hyperchromatic nuclei are relatively small and may actually be smaller than those seen in normal hepatocytes,

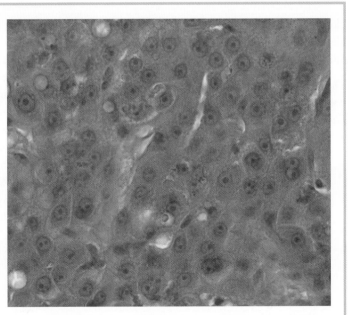

Figure 9.6
Liver biopsy showing nuclear crowding with cells with relatively small nuclei but with an increased nuclear:cytoplasmic ratio. These are the features of small cell dysplasia, which is more worrying than large cell dysplasia.

Index

N.B. References to 'hepatitis' imply 'chronic hepatitis' unless otherwise stated.